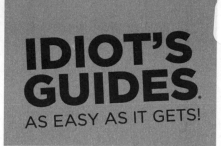

W9-BOO-326

Optimum Nutrition

by Stephanie Green, RDN

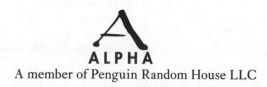

ALPHA

A member of Penguin Random House LLC

To my husband Duane—it's been a joy to share my life, love, and business with you.

ALPHA BOOKS

Published by Penguin Random House LLC

Penguin Random House LLC, 375 Hudson Street, New York, New York 10014, USA • Penguin Random House LLC (Canada), 90 Eglinton Avenue East, Suite 700, Toronto, Ontario M4P 2Y3, Canada (a division of Pearson Penguin Canada Inc.) • Penguin Books Ltd., 80 Strand, London WC2R 0RL, England • Penguin Ireland, 25 St. Stephen's Green, Dublin 2, Ireland (a division of Penguin Books Ltd.) • Penguin Random House LLC (Australia), 250 Camberwell Road, Camberwell, Victoria 3124, Australia (a division of Pearson Australia Group Pty. Ltd.) • Penguin Books India Pvt. Ltd., 11 Community Centre, Panchsheel Park, New Delhi—110 017, India • Penguin Random House LLC (NZ), 67 Apollo Drive, Rosedale, North Shore, Auckland 1311, New Zealand (a division of Pearson New Zealand Ltd.) • Penguin Books (South Africa) (Pty.) Ltd., 24 Sturdee Avenue, Rosebank, Johannesburg 2196, South Africa • Penguin Books Ltd., Registered Offices: 80 Strand, London WC2R 0RL, England

Copyright © 2015 by Penguin Random House LLC

001-289044-January2016

IDIOT'S GUIDES and Design are trademarks of Penguin Random House LLC

International Standard Book Number: 978-1-61564-8849
Library of Congress Catalog Card Number: 2015941382

17 16 15   8 7 6 5 4 3 2 1

Interpretation of the printing code: The rightmost number of the first series of numbers is the year of the book's printing; the rightmost number of the second series of numbers is the number of the book's printing. For example, a printing code of 15-1 shows that the first printing occurred in 2015.

Printed in the United States of America

Note: This publication contains the opinions and ideas of its author. It is intended to provide helpful and informative material on the subject matter covered. It is sold with the understanding that the author and publisher are not engaged in rendering professional services in the book. If the reader requires personal assistance or advice, a competent professional should be consulted. The author and publisher specifically disclaim any responsibility for any liability, loss, or risk, personal or otherwise, which is incurred as a consequence, directly or indirectly, of the use and application of any of the contents of this book.

Most Alpha books are available at special quantity discounts for bulk purchases for sales promotions, premiums, fundraising, or educational use. Special books, or book excerpts, can also be created to fit specific needs. For details, write: Special Markets, Alpha Books, 375 Hudson Street, New York, NY 10014.

Publisher: *Mike Sanders*
Associate Publisher: *Billy Fields*
Acquisitions Editor: *Jan Lynn*
Development Editor: *John Etchison*
Cover Designer: *Laura Merriman*

Book Designer: *William Thomas*
Indexer: *Celia McCoy*
Layout: *Ayanna Lacey*
Proofreader: *Amy Borrelli*

Contents

Introduction

We don't always get a chance for a "do over" in life, but when it comes to nutrition we can rebuild a better, stronger foundation for good health. If you're ready to take a proactive approach to your nutrition through practical, doable steps, this book can be your guide to optimum nutrition. It will broaden your understanding of the important roles of nutrients in the foods you eat and their impact on your health. We also provide food and lifestyle strategies to begin on your path toward better health.

Food is the key to good nutrition, but where do you begin? We're going to embark on this journey toward good nutrition one step at a time with very easy-to-understand segments. We provide you with the inner workings of nutrition—why nutrients are essential to good health, how your body uses them, and in what foods you'll find them. We give you tips for preparing nutritious meals regardless your lifestyle, and even include a few recipes to whet your appetite.

Sometimes simple dietary changes can help you feel better; other times more help is needed. We'll help you identify when it's time to seek professional help to get your body running smoothly and live a healthier, more active life.

This book was written to provide you with a thorough, easy-to-read, science-based background in nutrition and to serve as a reference for making positive nutrition changes in your life. We hope you enjoy it and start making strides toward better nutrition and health.

How This Book Is Organized

The chapters in this book are divided into five parts. Each part focuses on a certain aspect of nutrition and health.

Part 1, Nutrition and Wellness: An Overview, helps you understand your current state of nutrition and how to become healthier. We show you how to know if you're at risk and provide simple ways for improvement. We'll also explore the connection between food and mood.

Part 2, The Basics of Nutrition, provides you with the fascinating way nutrients are absorbed and digested. We examine the role of carbohydrates, proteins, and fats, along with vitamins, minerals, and plant-based nutrients, and how they work in your body to support vital functions and help ward off disease. We look at how much of these nutrients you need and the best sources to obtain them.

Part 3, Making Your Best Food Choices, explores all the major foods you need for good health, as well as how to avoid certain categories. We take an in-depth look at the best cooking oils for better health. We cover how food gets from farm to table and explain the differences between organic and conventionally grown produce. Finally, we teach you how to decipher food labels and understand health claims.

Part 4, Your Healthy Diet, shows you how to create a better way to cook and eat healthier. We also teach you how to listen to your body's food cues and deal with cravings. We give you the best ways to navigate through a restaurant menu to make healthy choices. And we explore the differences between food allergies, food sensitivities, and food intolerances and how to live with them.

In **Part 5, What Science Says About Special Foods,** we explore the top diets and their impact on your health. We also look at how certain foods are "super" in regards to health. We investigate how farms and ranches raise animals and what terms like cage-free and grain-fed really mean to the consumer.

Extras

Scattered throughout the book you'll notice sidebars that contain information to aid in your understanding of the subject matter.

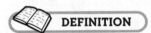

DEFINITION

These sidebars provide you with definitions of terms that are relevant to the topic.

FOODIE FACTOID

These sidebars present interesting food-related facts.

NOTABLE INSIGHT

These sidebars contain tips or direct you to more in-depth information you can find elsewhere.

WAKE-UP CALL

These sidebars contain health warnings or alerts you should be watchful for.

Acknowledgments

Thank you to my wonderful research assistant, Nona Bennett, RDN, who worked so diligently with me to pull this book together. Thanks for all of your long, hard work and your fantastic attitude. It was a pleasure working with you.

Thank you to my literary agent, Beth Campbell at BookEnds, LLC, for bringing this delightful project to me, and a very big thanks to editors Jan Lynn and John Etchison.

Many thanks to the nutrition professionals and dietetic interns from ASU and Maricopa County, who provided assistance on this project, and a big shout out to Chef Teresa Hansen for always lending a helping hand.

A special thank you to my husband, Duane, for all of his incredible support during the writing of this book. He took care of all of life's little details so that I could maintain my focus on this project. You're the best!

Trademarks

All terms mentioned in this book that are known to be or are suspected of being trademarks or service marks have been appropriately capitalized. Alpha Books and Penguin Random House LLC cannot attest to the accuracy of this information. Use of a term in this book should not be regarded as affecting the validity of any trademark or service mark.

Nutrition and Wellness: An Overview

You're probably one of the millions of people who are concerned about good nutrition. What is it? How do you achieve it? And yes, it's true: you are indeed what you eat. Good nutrition can be attained, but you've got to know where to start. However, before you begin, we need to lay down a solid foundation on which to build. This part will help identify where you are health-wise, and determine if you're already at risk. We'll also take a look at eating hazards, discuss how they lead to disease, and show you what you can do to avoid them.

Even though you have good intentions about eating healthy, your mind gets in the way sometimes and sabotages your plan. In this part, we examine the connection between food and mood, and review how foods can actually impact your mental health.

What Is Good Nutrition?

Good nutrition is the foundation to good health. It assures your body has the nutrients it needs to support growth and function optimally. When you eat a healthy, well-balanced diet, you maintain your weight, help ward off disease, gain mental clarity, and genuinely feel better.

In this chapter, we'll take a look at how you can make better food choices, what makes a well-balanced meal, and how exercise and stress affects well-being. Additionally, we'll do a quick risk assessment of your health.

In This Chapter

- A proactive approach to good health through nutrition
- Determining your health risk factors
- Tools to help you evaluate your diet
- How to filter the media hype around nutrition and health
- Exercise and its role in good health
- What are the components of a healthy lifestyle?

How to Get Healthy

Good nutrition is the gateway to good health, but being really healthy involves a whole life approach. You need to take a proactive approach toward your health and not wait until a health issue is present before taking an active role in your well-being. Getting healthy means making good food choices, participating in an active lifestyle, finding ways to alleviate stress, and maintaining a joyful outlook on life. All of these things work in unison to make for a long and healthy life.

Eat Good Foods

Eating good foods sounds easy, right? So why isn't everyone eating healthy? Well, it's not so simple, especially if you've spent a lifetime learning poor eating habits. You may have to redefine what makes a healthy meal and seek out those foods, some of which may be new to you. Overhauling your diet can seem like an overwhelming task, but it doesn't have to be. Some people can get started on their own and others need a little guidance and support. But before you can make a change in your eating pattern, you need to know what you've been doing wrong. This will give you a way to evaluate where you are and the areas you need to work on.

An easy way to begin the process is to keep a food log. A food log is a record of what you ate or drank, and the specific time and day you ate or drank it. Keeping track for about a week will provide you with a good picture of what you've been eating and the types of foods that dominate your diet. Next, evaluate how you're doing by asking yourself the following questions as you review your food log:

- Are 50 percent of your meals made up of fruits and vegetables?

- Are the majority of your grains from whole grain sources?

- What percentage of added fats are present in your meals? Less than 10 percent?

- Do 25 percent of each of your main meals (breakfast, lunch, and dinner) contain lean protein sources?

- What percentage of foods are from sugary and refined snacks? Less than 10 percent?

- Do you have three servings of dairy each day?

- Do you eat three meals a day, along with snacks?

Most people have room for improvement, and it's important to gradually make small changes in your diet. One way to begin is to add more fruit and vegetables. Decide on a goal such as the addition of one fruit or vegetable per day for the entire week. It should be something you enjoy eating, too. There's no point in making unrealistic goals, such as starting your day with a glowing green smoothie made of dandelion greens, kale, carrot, ginger, and an apple, when you don't own a blender and you don't even know if you like dandelion greens! An easy solution would be to add more vegetables you're already familiar with to your diet.

Good nutrition involves a variety of nutrient-dense foods. We can classify them into five food groups. Each group provides a variety of essential vitamins, minerals, and plant nutrients like phytochemicals to help keep your body strong and healthy and help ward off disease. The five food groups are fruits, vegetables, grains, protein, and dairy. Your total number of servings varies based on your age, sex, and activity level. Check out the following table for specific recommendations based on your age and gender.

What's a general serving size?

- Fruit: 1 cup of fruit, 1 cup of 100% fruit juice, or ½ cup of dried fruit

- Vegetables: 1 cup of raw or cooked vegetables, 1 cup of 100% vegetable juice, or 2 cups of leafy greens

- Whole grains: 1 slice of bread; 1 cup of dry cereal; or ½ cup of cooked cereal, rice, or pasta

- Protein: 1 ounce of meat, poultry, or fish; ¼ cup of beans; 1 egg; 1 tablespoon of peanut butter; or ½ ounce of nuts or seeds

- Dairy: 1 cup of dairy milk, yogurt, or soymilk; 1½ ounces of natural cheese; 2 ounces of processed cheese

Foods	Number of Servings per Day					
	Women Age Range			Men Age Range		
	19-30	31-50	51+	19-30	31-50	51+
Fruit	2 cups	1.5 cups	1.5 cups	2 cups	2 cups	2 cups
Vegetables	2.5 cups	2.5 cups	2 cups	3 cups	3 cups	2.5 cups
Whole Grains	6 oz.	6 oz.	5 oz.	8 oz.	7 oz.	6 oz.
Protein	5.5 oz.	5 oz.	5 oz.	6.5 oz.	6 oz.	5.5 oz.
Dairy	3 cups	3 cups	3 cups	3 cups	3 cups	3 cups
Fat	6 tsp.	5 tsp.	5 tsp.	7 tsp.	6 tsp.	6 tsp.

Serving recommendations based on choosemyplate.gov.

Get Moving

One of the key components to good health is exercise. For many people, exercise brings up overwhelming thoughts of going to a crowded, sweaty gym with lots of eyes judging you for being so out of shape. I'm here to tell you to stop playing that tape in your head and making excuses. Exercise doesn't have to be a negative. The benefits of just a little bit of exercise are astounding—from greater mental clarity to increased energy and improved sleep, just for starters.

The easiest way to add exercise into your life is to schedule a time to go for a walk. All you need is a good pair of walking shoes that provide adequate support and stability. Begin with a 5-minute walk if that's all the time or energy you have, and then when you're ready, push it to 10 minutes and so on. Ideally, your goal should be 30 minutes per day for heart health, according to the American Heart Association (AHA).

Next, you need to begin to monitor your heart rate. Your target heart rate should be between 50 and 70 percent of your maximum heart rate. The simplest way to tell is if you can still carry on a conversation while you're exercising; if you can't, your heart rate is too high. Keeping your heart rate in the "zone" helps you burn more calories.

 NOTABLE INSIGHT

Exercise doesn't have to equate to running. It can be anything that gets you moving. Check out the calories burned based on a person who weighs 155 pounds and is active for 30 minutes:

- Walking 4 mph: 167 calories
- Swimming: 223 calories
- Raking the lawn: 149 calories
- Gardening: 167 calories
- Cooking: 93 calories
- Food shopping w/cart: 130 calories

Data from the Harvard Heart Letter *from Harvard Medical School.*

To determine your target heart rate, you must first find out what your resting heart rate is. According to the National Institutes of Health (NIH), the average resting heart rate is between 60 and 100 beats per minute for adults.

How to take your pulse:

- Using the tips of your index and middle finger, place them lightly on the opposite wrist on the inside just down from your thumb. Do this first thing in the morning before you get out of bed to get a more accurate result.

- Count the beats for 10 seconds and multiply by 6 to find your beats per minute. Write that number down. If you're in the average resting heart rate zone, then calculate your maximum heart rate. If your resting heart rate is above average, you should speak with your doctor as soon as possible.

- Calculate your maximum heart rate by subtracting your age from 220. For example, 220 - 35 years old = 185 maximum heart rate.

Now multiply your maximum heart rate by 0.5 (50 percent) to determine the lower end of your target heart rate zone: $185 \times 0.5 = 92.5$

Next calculate the upper level of your target heart rate range by multiplying by 0.7.

$185 \times 0.7 = 129.5$ or 70 percent of your maximum heart rate

Your range of 92.5–129.5 (or 93–130) is your target zone.

If you haven't exercised in a long time, it's a good idea to start out by keeping your target heart rate at 50 percent and then increase your range as you get more fit. However, before you start any exercise program, it's a good idea to check with your doctor and also keep in mind that some medications can alter your heart rate.

Manage Your Stress

Eating regular nutrient-rich meals can help alleviate stress, especially if they contain foods high in omega-3 fatty acids like salmon and flaxseeds, which have been proven to help even out the body's stress hormones. See Chapter 8 for a list of foods high in omega-3s. There are also other ways to help manage your stress utilizing techniques like *meditation* and exercise.

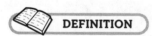 **DEFINITION**

> **Meditation** is a practice that helps you find inner peace. It also helps you deal with life stress and has been used for centuries as a way to calm the body. Follow these simple tips to get started today:
>
> 1. Find a quiet place.
> 2. Get into a comfortable position either lying down or sitting.
> 3. Focus on a word or phrase that's soothing.
> 4. Observe your thoughts as they pass but redirect attention on your focus word or phrase.

Here are some tips to reduce stress:

- When feeling stressed, take three long deep breaths.

- Go easy on caffeinated beverages and alcohol.

- Eat nutrient-dense meals on a regular schedule.

- Get enough sleep each night.

- Exercise daily.

- Schedule downtime to really relax with stress-reducing activities such as meditating, journaling, or reading.

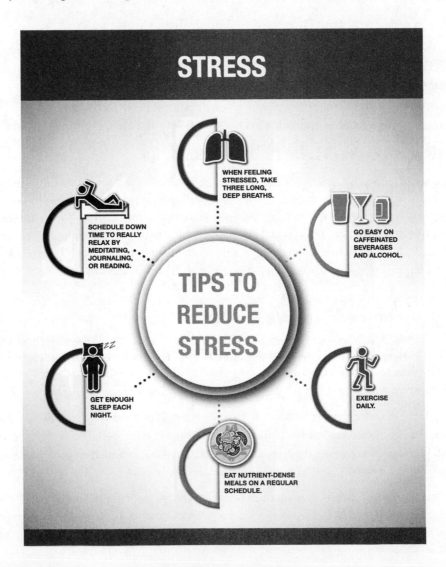

Is Your Health at Risk?

America is suffering from an epidemic of overweight and obesity, and the outlook doesn't seem to show signs of improvement. Weighing too much or being obese can lead to many diseases such as diabetes, heart disease, and some cancers. How can you tell if you are at risk? You need to know your numbers:

- **Know your BMI:** If it's greater than 25, you're overweight

- **Waist size:** Women >35 inches or men >40 inches are at greater health risk.

- **Blood pressure:** Should be 120/80 mmHg or less.

- **LDL "bad" cholesterol:** Should be less than 100mg/dL.

- **HDL "good" cholesterol:** More than 40mg/dL women and 50mg/dL men.

- **Triglycerides:** Should be less than 150mg/dL.

- **Fasting blood sugar:** Should be less than 100mg/dL.

The Keys to Good Nutrition

Nutrition is key to good health because it impacts your whole body and mental status. Not only does it help your body grow and repair itself, it has the potential to make corrections when cells go awry, especially those that can lead to cancer. Nutrition is so important, but unfortunately many people don't make it a priority until they're facing a health crisis.

Your approach to good nutrition should be through good foods. You must strive for variety and balance. The kinds of foods you want to build your nutrition base around are mostly derived from plants such as vegetables, fruits, and whole grains. If 75 percent of your diet is from these sources, you're headed in the right direction. Next, you would fill in the remaining 25 percent with animal-based proteins and dairy or dairy alternatives. This will automatically help you limit convenience and fast foods because you will be so well fed. By eating this way, you'll feel better, and have more energy and improved mental clarity. This is not to say that you shouldn't indulge a little every now and then, but it's important to know what you're putting into your body.

Reading labels and ingredient lists is vital when you want to focus on creating a healthy diet. You may discover your favorite "go to" food is full of the worst kind of fat and over the top in sodium content. Once you know the facts, the food may not be so appealing anymore. This is where making a rational, informed decision can lead to new eating habits that are better for your health.

Furthermore, good nutrition is about making this new way of eating a lifestyle and moving away from the diet mentality. It's about making small changes that can last a lifetime. Having the nutrition knowledge is one thing, but putting it into action is what matters most when it comes to your health.

The Dietary Guidelines for Americans

Every five years the U.S. government publishes the Dietary Guidelines for Americans. This is a joint effort between the U.S. Department of Health and Human Services (HHS) and the U.S. Department of Agriculture (USDA). These guidelines provide valuable information on what we should be eating and drinking to promote health, maintain our weight, and ward off health-related diseases like heart disease for all Americans over 2 years of age.

The first edition of Dietary Guidelines was released in 1980, and it reflected scientific evidence about diet and health. In 1985, they established a committee consisting of nutrition and health experts, which they have continued to do with each release. These committee members are appointed with each edition. Subcommittees and workgroups are established and public comments and meetings are held to discuss the relevant issues related to health and nutrition. Visit cnpp.usda.gov/DietaryGuidelines for the latest information.

While the 2015 recommendations haven't been released as of this book's writing, the key recommendations from the 2010 Dietary Guidelines for Americans on foods and food components to reduce in the diet are as follows:

- Reduce sodium to 2,300mg or if you are 51 and older, 1,500mg. If you are African American (any age) or have hypertension, diabetes, or chronic kidney disease, reduce your sodium intake to 1,500mg.

- Consume less than 10 percent of your calories from saturated fat and replace the saturated fat in your diet with monounsaturated and polyunsaturated fatty acids.

- Consume less than 300mg of cholesterol per day.

- Consume little to no trans fats, such as partially hydrogenated oils and solid fats.

- Reduce your intake of solid fats and added sugars.

- Limit your consumption of refined grains and those with added saturated fats, sodium, and sugar.

- Consume alcohol in moderation, up to one drink per day for women and two for men.

The foods and nutrients to increase in your daily diet are as follows:

- Increase vegetable and fruit intake by eating a variety of vegetables, especially dark-green, red, and orange vegetables, and beans and peas.

- Consume half of all your grains as whole grains and replace refined grains with whole ones.

- Increase your intake of fat-free or low-fat milk and milk products.

- Choose a variety of protein foods like seafood, lean meats, poultry, eggs, beans and peas, soy products, unsalted nuts, and seeds.

- Increase your amount and variety of seafood by replacing some meat and poultry items in your diet.

- Replace protein foods higher in solid fats with those that are lower in fat and calories.

- Use mono- and polyunsaturated vegetable oils to replace solid fats.

- Choose foods that provide more potassium, fiber, calcium, and vitamin D.

The Dietary Guidelines also includes specific recommendations for certain population groups. For instance, women who are thinking of becoming pregnant or are pregnant or breastfeeding should:

- Choose foods high in heme iron and vitamin C–rich foods and eat them at the same meal to enhance iron absorption.

- Take an iron supplement if pregnant.

- Consume 400mcg per day of synthetic folic acid from a supplement.

- Consume 8 to 12 ounces of seafood per week from a variety of sources.

- Limit seafood sources high in methyl mercury like white (albacore) tuna to 6 ounces per week and avoid tilefish, shark, swordfish, and king mackerel.

Additionally, those age 50 and older should eat foods fortified with B_{12} or are advised to take a dietary supplement.

Finding a Nutrition Expert and Support

Working with a nutritionist is a great way to help you improve your diet and reach your health goals. Nutritionists can point you in the right direction, keep you on track, and hold you accountable for your actions. They can also make sure you don't go overboard when trying to make too many changes at once. Most nutritionists specialize in certain areas such as weight loss, food allergies, food coaching, sports nutrition, diabetes, and eating disorders. It's a good idea to find one that's experienced in working with people with your specific health issues. Secondly, you need to feel really comfortable with this person, as food is quite personal.

It's important to realize that there is no legal definition associated with the word "nutritionist," so be sure to ask questions to determine the person's qualifications. Here are a few tips:

- Do they have a degree from a credible university?

- Have they completed a supervised practice program?

- Did they pass a national exam?

- Does their organization require continuing professional education?

A *registered dietitian nutritionist (RDN)* meets these qualifications and can be found all over the United States and the world.

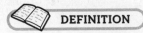

> **DEFINITION**
>
> A **registered dietitian nutritionist (RDN)** translates the science of nutrition into practical solutions for health. RDNs have a minimum of a Bachelor's degree in science, completed an accredited supervised practice program 6 to 12 months in length, passed a national examination, and are required to meet additional professional education requirements to maintain registration. There are over 70,000 RDNs worldwide. To find a RDN near you, go to eatright.org/find-an-expert.

The Least You Need to Know

- Eating healthy well-balanced meals that include the five major food groups can prevent certain health-related diseases.
- A food log is a great tool to evaluate your eating patterns.
- A variety of nutrient-dense foods, physical activity, and a good mental outlook can lead to good health and longevity.
- Selecting a nutritionist is a personal decision.

You Are What You Eat

The foods we put in our bodies every day go a long way to determine the state of our health. Foods are chockfull of vitamins, minerals, and other essential nutrients the body needs to maintain proper functioning and energy levels, as well as decrease our risk for chronic disease. It's like the old adage, if you put bad gas in a car it won't run correctly. Well, if you put bad foods in your body, it, too, won't run properly. At some point, your body will stall, leaving you at risk for many types of health issues.

In this chapter, we'll provide you with the reasons that you are indeed what you eat. You'll discover how foods can lead to health hazards and how others may be part of the solution. Not only is it what you eat that can affect your health, but your overall lifestyle in addition to something you have no control over—family genetics.

In This Chapter

- Obesity and preventable deaths
- Foods with a negative impact on health
- Foods that help to prevent or manage common health problems
- Your lifestyle and your risk for chronic diseases

The Road to Good Health

Unfortunately for us, there's no one magic food that will put us on the fast track to good health. The key is to consume a variety of healthy foods each day and to live a healthy lifestyle. If family genetics is a concern, a healthy diet and lifestyle become even more imperative if you intend to keep traveling down the right road. The goal is to take care of your body, both inside and out, in order to decrease your risk for health issues such as obesity, heart disease, cancer, and diabetes, just to name a few.

Sometimes the road to good health can seem like a juggling act, but the trick is to turn it into a balancing act. It doesn't need to be difficult, but it does take some effort. You need to balance eating right, exercising, getting plenty of sleep, and de-stressing whenever possible. Sounds easy, right?

You should start by including a good doctor on your team, one that focuses on wellness and is proactive. Be sure you get a full checkup on a yearly basis. Next, learn all you can about good nutrition and put it into practice. There are plenty of resources to help, including the United States Department of Agriculture's (USDA) ChooseMyPlate.gov and the Dietary Guidelines for Americans, not to mention all the good information in this book. Start by adopting healthier habits such as exercise and healthy eating, and the rest will fall into place!

 NOTABLE INSIGHT

Both ChooseMyPlate.gov and the Dietary Guidelines for Americans (cnpp.usda.gov/ DietaryGuidelines) are issued and updated jointly by the Department of Agriculture (USDA) and the Department of Health and Human Services (HHS) every 5 years. Both guidelines work hand-in-hand to provide the most current science-based advice for all Americans 2 years and older. They're available so that we can educate ourselves as to what good nutrition is and how we can make healthier choices. The key is not to only read both of these educational components, but to implement them in your everyday life.

Eating Hazards and Solutions for Health Issues

The foods and beverages you choose to consume can either be a hazard to your health or the solution to better overall health. The choice is yours! It's up to you to feed your body foods that help and protect rather than injure. Whether you have a health issue or not, it's in your best interest to consume foods that will improve your overall health and decrease your risk for chronic disease. The foods you choose to consume are something you have complete control over and a change you can start immediately.

There are many health issues that can be directly related to the foods we consume. On the other hand, there are foods that can also help to prevent and/or manage certain health issues. We'll visit some of the more common health issues that plague Americans, and discover which foods can create a hazard and which can be the solution.

Obesity

It's well known that obesity is a major problem in our country, but do you realize what it can do to your body and your health? Obesity-related conditions include heart disease, stroke, type 2 diabetes, and some types of cancer, just to name a few. All of these health issues are the leading causes of preventable deaths. In other words, reaching and maintaining a healthy body weight can prevent or help lower your risk for many of these types of health issues.

NOTABLE INSIGHT

According to the Centers for Disease Control and Prevention (CDC), more than one third of the adult population in the United States is obese.

For many people obesity is directly related to food and beverages, mainly the types chosen in addition to portion sizes and calories consumed. This, in conjunction with a poor activity level, can and usually does lead to obesity.

Here are ways to begin to address your weight issues:

- Assess your weight using the Body Mass Index (BMI), which can tell you if you're at a healthy weight. See Chapter 5 for more information on BMI and assessing your weight.

- If you're not at a healthy weight, take steps to lose weight. Just a modest amount of weight loss, 5 to 10 percent of your current weight, can make a positive impact on your health.

- Slow and steady weight loss is the most successful way to lose weight and keep it off. It's all about an ongoing lifestyle change in daily eating and exercise habits.

- To lose weight, you need to burn more calories than you consume. Since 1 pound equals 3,500 calories, reduce your caloric intake by 500 to 1,000 calories per day for a safe and recommended rate of weight loss of 1 to 2 pounds per week.

- If you rely on a healthful diet and regular exercise to lose weight, your chances for success in both the long and the short term will be very good.

Eating the wrong types of foods and/or eating too much of them can tip the scales in the wrong direction, putting you at risk for obesity and therefore a host of health problems. This is not to say that eating these foods will definitely lead to obesity, but if eaten in large quantities on a regular basis, chances are you'll head down that road. Any food, unhealthy or healthy, can lead to excess weight gain if you eat too much of it. It's all about balance and moderation!

Hazard foods that can lead to obesity include:

- **Fast food:** These foods contain mostly unhealthy fats, too much sodium, and large amounts of calories. Fast food on a regular basis can cause obesity and all sorts of health issues.

- **High-sugar foods:** Examples are candy; baked goods such as cookies, cakes, pies, and donuts; table sugar; and sugar-sweetened beverages such as soda, sports drinks, energy drinks, and bottled iced teas. These foods contain way too much sugar and too many calories, and have no nutritional value. Eating them on a regular basis will lead to weight gain.

- **Alcohol:** Too much alcohol can add too many unnecessary calories to your diet and leave less room for healthy foods.

- **Refined or processed grains:** These foods include white breads, sugary cereals, white rice, and other foods made with white flour. They lack the fiber and nutritional value of whole grains and other healthier carbs. In addition, they make you hungrier more quickly and can cause overeating, which leads to obesity.

- **High-fat foods:** These include foods full of saturated fats such as full-fat dairy products, some salad dressings, and fatty or processed meats. They add unhealthy fats along with too many calories to your diet.

 NOTABLE INSIGHT

A study published in *The American Journal of Clinical Nutrition* involving 19,352 Swedish women who consumed one to two whole-fat dairy products daily showed that there was an inverse relationship to weight gain. This may be because the whole-fat products provided increased satiety levels, which led to eating less later on, or the fact that some of the fatty acids may play a role in weight regulation.

Eating the right types of foods in moderate portions can help you reach and/or maintain a healthy weight. It will also lower your risk for many chronic diseases since these foods are also good for your health.

Solution foods that can help prevent obesity include:

- **A variety of fruits and vegetables:** These foods add nutritional value, healthy calories, and fiber to meals and snacks.

- **Whole-grains:** Foods such as whole-wheat bread, brown rice, oatmeal, and quinoa add fiber and nutritional value to help fill you up quicker and keep your energy and blood sugar levels more stable.

- **Nuts, seeds, and beans:** These foods add healthy fats, protein, and nutritional value to your diet.

- **Fish, seafood, and lean meats:** These lean protein sources help to satisfy your hunger when included in a well-balanced meal.

- **Unsaturated fats:** Foods containing fats such as plant oils and avocados add health benefits and satiety to meals.

 WAKE-UP CALL

Fad diets may seem like the easy and quick way to lose weight, but don't be in such a hurry. Most fad diets are just that, "diets" that are a temporary fix to a lifelong problem. Fad diets can lead to nutritional deficiencies, metabolic issues, and muscle loss. Most don't work, and definitely don't work long-term. Some rely on supplements that contain caffeine, other stimulants, and harmful chemicals. You should steer clear of fad diets.

Heart Disease

Heart disease, such as coronary heart disease, heart attack, stroke, and congestive heart failure, is currently the leading cause of death for both men and women in the United States. Lowering your risk for heart disease includes eating healthier foods, exercising, maintaining a healthy weight, quitting smoking, managing your blood pressure, and lowering blood cholesterol levels. Although some heart issues can be genetic, lifestyle habits do play a major role in both preventing and managing heart disease.

There are plenty of foods that are directly involved with many of the risk factors for heart disease. Paying close attention to what you eat is one of the most important preventative measures you can take to help protect your heart.

Hazard foods that can increase your risk for heart disease include:

- **Saturated fat:** Foods that contain saturated fat include butter, sour cream, mayonnaise, and fatty cuts of meat, especially red meats. Saturated fat can increase your "bad" blood cholesterol levels, as well as the risk for heart attack.

- **Trans fat:** Foods that contain hydrogenated oil or partially hydrogenated oil contain trans fat. These fats lower your "good" cholesterol and raise your "bad" cholesterol. Big culprits include packaged snacks, crackers, baked goods, and some margarines. Always read labels carefully to ensure you're avoiding trans fats. The Food and Drug Administration (FDA) ruled in June 2015 for all trans fats to be removed from food products.

- **High-sodium foods:** Too much sodium in the diet can lead to high blood pressure for some people, which is a major risk factor for heart disease.

- **Added sugars:** Added sugars are the sugar added to foods by consumers or manufacturers. High added sugar intakes may be linked with high blood sugar and high triglyceride levels, both of which are risk factors for heart disease.

Solution foods that can help prevent heart disease include:

- **Fruits and vegetables:** These foods are full of antioxidants and fiber, which are both heart friendly.

- **Sources of vitamin E:** This vitamin may help protect against "bad" cholesterol, and therefore help protect the heart. Foods containing vitamin E include nuts, leafy greens, fortified whole-grains, avocados, and vegetable oils.

- **Fatty fish:** Fish such as mackerel, sardines, tuna, and salmon contain omega-3 fatty acids, which have been shown to be heart healthy.

- **Healthy fats:** These fats include monounsaturated and polyunsaturated fat in foods such as olive oil, canola oil, certain fish, nuts, seeds, and avocados. Unsaturated fats, when used in place of saturated fats, help lower cholesterol levels and therefore the risk of heart disease.

FOODIE FACTOID

An easy way to add heart-healthy fats and fiber to your diet is to add ground flaxseed to your foods. Flaxseed is high in both fiber and omega-3 fatty acids as well as antioxidants and lignans. Ground flaxseed is more absorbable than whole seeds. It can help lower cholesterol levels as well as help improve blood sugar levels, and works as an anti-inflammatory. You can add 1 to 2 tablespoons of ground flaxseed daily to smoothies, nonfat yogurt, hot cereal, mashed potatoes, etc. Flaxseed is usually not recommended during pregnancy and is categorized as "possibly unsafe" according to the National Institutes of Health (NIH) due to the possible estrogren-like effects; however, there is no reliable clinical evidence at this time regarding effects on pregnancy.

Type 2 Diabetes

Type 2 diabetes is a metabolic disorder in which the body is unable to produce enough insulin or unable to use it effectively. It causes your blood glucose (sugar) levels to rise higher than they normally should be. Glucose in your blood comes from the digestion of carbohydrates and is an essential form of sugar your body uses for energy. However, too much blood sugar can be harmful and do plenty of damage to your body.

Food is a major component to preventing and managing type 2 diabetes. Being overweight or obese is a major risk factor. In addition, what you eat, including sugars and carbohydrates, will affect your blood sugar levels. There are foods that can be hazards and ones that can be solutions.

Hazard foods that can increase your risk for type 2 diabetes include:

- **Refined grains and foods made mostly with white flour:** These include white breads, white rice, white pasta, and sugary cereals. They usually have a higher *glycemic index (GI)*, and therefore are broken down quickly into sugar, making controlling blood sugar more difficult.

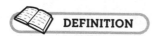

DEFINITION

Glycemic index (GI) is a measurement of how much each gram of available carbohydrate (total carbohydrate minus fiber) in a single serving of a food affects your blood sugar level.

- **Sweetened foods and beverages:** Any food or beverage with added sugars derived from any source could provide a sugar load to your system and may increase *insulin resistance.* It also provides excess calories, which can lead to weight gain.

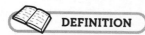

DEFINITION

Insulin resistance occurs when the body can produce insulin without a problem but cannot utilize it effectively. Body cells don't respond properly to insulin, and therefore cannot absorb glucose from the bloodstream, resulting in the body needing higher levels of insulin for glucose to enter the cells.

- **Fruit juices:** Who knew that fruit juice could be a problem for diabetics? Juice can cause sharp spikes in blood sugar for people with diabetes due to its concentrated source of fruit sugar and lack of fiber. If the juice isn't "100 percent juice," it contains loads of added sugars as well. Whole fruit is a much better option.

- **Whole-fat dairy products:** Dairy products are important; however, choosing the right types is even more important. Whole-fat dairy products are loaded with saturated fats because they're an animal product, and those fats can worsen insulin resistance, which is the last thing a person with diabetes needs. Fill your refrigerator with fat-free or low-fat dairy counterparts such as fat-free milk, low-fat cheese, and low-fat yogurts.

Solution foods that can help prevent and manage type 2 diabetes include:

- **High-soluble fiber foods:** Soluble fiber can help slow the absorption of glucose (or blood sugar) from the food in our stomach and help better control blood sugar levels over time. Foods high in soluble fiber include oatmeal, oat bran, apples, oranges, pears, strawberries, blueberries, lentils, nuts, flaxseeds, beans, carrots, cucumbers, and psyllium.

- **Monounsaturated fats:** These are healthy fats and are great for overall health. When it comes to diabetes, however, studies have shown that a diet high in monounsaturated fats and low in refined carbohydrates may help to improve insulin resistance and control blood sugar. Monounsaturated foods include avocados, almonds and other nuts, olive oil, and canola oil.

- **Berries:** All fruit is part of a healthy diet, but berries in particular (such as blueberries, strawberries, blackberries, and raspberries), due to their powerful antioxidant content, have been shown to reduce the risk for certain health issues including type 2 diabetes. Blackberries are particularly high in fiber, which is also helpful in managing diabetes. Blueberries contain specific antioxidant compounds that have antidiabetic properties and may help to improve insulin resistance.

- **Whole-grains:** Made with whole grains, these foods include whole-wheat breads, oatmeal, brown rice, whole-grain pasta, quinoa, and bulgur. They're full of vitamins, minerals, phytonutrients, and fiber. They're a steadier source of energy and help to keep blood sugar levels more stable.

Hypertension

Hypertension may not ring a bell, but I'm sure you've heard of high blood pressure. Hypertension is just a fancier name for this common condition. In fact, one in four Americans has been diagnosed with hypertension. Blood pressure is the force of blood against the artery walls as the heart pumps blood through the body. Blood pressure that's consistently high can eventually cause blood vessel damage and health issues such as heart disease, kidney disease, and stroke. Because hypertension has minor or no symptoms, it can be a silent killer. Many people can go years without even realizing they have it unless a doctor checks for it. However, by then the damage often is already done.

Blood pressure readings are given as two numbers, systolic (the top number) and diastolic (the bottom number). Blood pressure levels lower than 120/80 mmHg indicate normal blood pressure. However, if you have known heart or kidney issues or have had a stroke, your pressure may need to be lower than normal. High blood pressure or hypertension is when blood pressure is higher than 140/90 mmHg.

Just like other health issues, food can play a major role in both preventing and managing hypertension. As far as hypertension goes, your best bet is to do all you can to prevent it from occurring in the first place.

Hazard foods that can increase your risk for hypertension include:

- **Sodium:** Many people are sodium sensitive, and therefore too much sodium in their diet can lead to high blood pressure. Since it's difficult to know if you're one of these people, it's best to control your sodium intake to help prevent high blood pressure. If you already have high blood pressure, it's important to limit the amount of sodium you consume. Most sodium in our diet comes from processed and packaged foods, fast foods, and table salt. The American Heart Association (AHA) recommends consuming less than 1,500 milligrams of sodium per day.

- **Alcohol:** Drinking too much alcohol can cause high blood pressure. If you do drink, limit your alcohol intake to no more than two drinks per day for men and one drink per day for women to help prevent or manage high blood pressure.

- **Low potassium:** This mineral is essential for allowing the smooth muscle cells in your arteries to relax, which lowers blood pressure. When your potassium intake is low, you can be putting yourself at risk for hypertension.

- **Low vitamin D:** There's a possibility that too little vitamin D in your diet can increase your risk for high blood pressure. Researchers believe vitamin D may affect a certain enzyme produced by your kidneys that affects blood pressure. While more studies need to be done, it's definitely a plus to ensure you're getting plenty of vitamin D in your diet by including fatty fish as well as fortified dairy products.

Solution foods that can help prevent and manage hypertension include:

- **Calcium-rich foods:** It has been found that populations with low calcium intake have higher rates of hypertension. This isn't to say you need to get more than what is generally recommended, but there may be some protective effects if you get the recommended daily intake of calcium, preferably through food. Good sources include low-fat and fat-free dairy foods, dark-green leafy veggies, canned salmon, calcium-fortified foods such as soy foods and orange juice, and almonds. The recommended intake is 1,000 to 1,200 mg/day.

- **Fruits and veggies:** A higher consumption of fruits and vegetables is associated with a lower risk of hypertension. Eating a variety of fruits (especially citrus fruits, tomatoes, and bananas) daily, as well as leafy greens and root vegetables such as potatoes and carrots, is a great way to ensure you're getting plenty of potassium daily.

- **Fatty fish:** This fish is high in good fat; omega-3 fatty acids; and includes salmon, mackerel, herring, lake trout, sardines, and albacore tuna. Research has shown that omega-3 fatty acids can have a positive impact on blood pressure. The AHA recommends eating a serving of fish (3.5 ounces cooked), especially fatty fish, at least twice per week.

- **Garlic:** You may love to cook with it, but it offers more than just flavor. Currently garlic is being researched to uncover possible benefits to lowering blood pressure.

 FOODIE FACTOID

Fruits are helpful in the fight against hypertension, but it appears that berries of all kinds, such as blueberries, strawberries, raspberries, and blackberries, are especially rich in a compound called flavonoids, which might help prevent high blood pressure and even reduce blood pressure that's already high.

Cancer

Unfortunately, just about all of us know someone who has had cancer. In fact, according to the American Cancer Society, 1 million people are diagnosed with cancer in the United States each year. Fortunately, there are steps we can take to decrease our risk, including not smoking, maintaining a healthy weight, eating healthy, staying active, and getting the recommended screening tests.

Hazard foods that can increase your risk for certain types of cancer include:

- **Salted, pickled, and smoked foods:** These types of foods, as well as some processed meats such as hot dogs, commonly contain additives called nitrates. These nitrates may have a cancer-causing effect.

- **Trans fat:** As we discussed earlier, trans fats are another component of some foods that again comes with several links to health problems. It's one of the worst fats you can eat and has been linked to certain types of cancer. Your best bet is to stay away from it altogether. In June 2015, the FDA ruled that all food manufacturers eliminate it completely over the next three years.

- **Charred foods:** Although cooking on the grill can be a great way to cook without fat, you still need to be careful. That well-done, charred burger can contain cancer-causing compounds. Try marinating your meat first, cut down the time and temperature at which the meat is cooked, and cut off charred spots. If you cook meat at high temps on the stove, use peanut oil, which can best handle the heat.

Solution foods that can help prevent cancer include:

- **Vitamin C-rich foods:** Vitamin C is a powerful antioxidant that can help lower your risk for cancer. Rich sources of vitamin C include grapefruit, oranges, bell peppers, and broccoli. Stick with vitamin C from foods as opposed to taking a supplement.

- **Berries:** Berries seem to pop up quite a bit as a solution food to many health issues, including cancer. Berries, especially blueberries, contain an antioxidant called pterostilbene that has cancer-fighting properties. Berries in general contain loads of cancer-fighting phytonutrients.

- **Sweet potatoes:** Sweet potatoes, in addition to other foods that contain large amounts of beta-carotene, have cancer-fighting effects. Beta-carotene is a powerful antioxidant grouped into carotenoids that gives some plant foods their color. Foods high in beta-carotene include mostly orange vegetables, such as sweet potatoes and carrots, as well as leafy greens.

- **Wild salmon:** This fish is rich in vitamin D, which is important because low levels of vitamin D intake have been linked to certain types of cancer. Salmon also contains the healthy omega-3 fatty acids.

 FOODIE FACTOID

Salmon doesn't naturally produce omega-3s. It comes from what the fish eats. Salmon eat herring, anchovies, and mackerel, otherwise referred to as "feeder" fish.

Inflammation

We're not talking about the occasional inflammation in your knee or the cut you had that became inflamed. We're talking about chronic inflammation. This type of inflammation can last from several months to years, and plays a bit of a puzzling role in the body. When inflammation becomes chronic, it affects healthy tissue and can become the root problem to all types of health issues, including asthma, arthritis, lupus, heart disease, certain types of cancer, and type 2 diabetes.

Food is a large part of helping to reduce and/or eliminate chronic inflammation. Experts believe that anti-inflammatory benefits come from the synergistic effect of foods that are consumed together as well as from individual foods.

Hazard foods that can increase your risk for inflammation include:

- **Red meat:** Most of us love that sizzling steak, but a 2014 study in *The American Journal of Clinical Nutrition* found that greater red meat intake is associated with unfavorable plasma concentrations of inflammatory biomarkers. Substituting red meat with other sources of healthier protein foods is associated with a lower biomarker profile of inflammation. The solution is to decrease your intake of red meats as much as possible.

- **Alcohol:** Regular consumption of alcohol can have negative health effects that range from heart disease to insulin resistance, all of which can increase and/or cause chronic inflammation. Keep in mind moderation: no more than two drinks per day for men and one per day for women.

- **High-sugar snacks and beverages:** There's a definite overconsumption of high-sugar foods and drinks in our country, which may explain some of the health problems that plague people in the United States. Excess sugar leads to weight gain and can cause spikes in both blood sugar and insulin, which in turn can trigger chronic inflammation.

- **Sodium:** Sodium is an essential mineral we need in our body for some very vital functions. However, when we consume too much sodium, not only can it cause high blood pressure for those who are sodium sensitive, but it can exacerbate inflammatory conditions such as arthritis.

Solution foods that can help decrease your risk for chronic inflammation include:

- **Dark-green leafy vegetables:** Most vegetables contain a wide variety of phytonutrients, including flavonoids (quercitin) and carotenoids (lutein and beta-carotene), but dark-green leafy vegetables such as spinach, kale, and collard greens are at the top of the list in terms of their specific content. These specific veggies have more than a dozen different flavonoid compounds that function as anti-inflammatory and anticancer agents as well as antioxidants.

- **Tart cherries:** This fruit contains a very potent class of flavonoids called anthocyanins. Anthocyanins are what give cherries, berries, and other fruits and vegetables their deep, rich colors. Cherries are an anthocyanin-rich food that delivers substantial antioxidant properties and anti-inflammatory activity and can help relieve pain by working in much the same way aspirin and nonsteroidal anti-inflammatory drugs do. Both tart cherries and sweet cherries have high concentrations of anthocyanins; however, tart cherries such as Balaton and Montmorency varieties contain the highest content and also contain other supporting compounds.

- **Ginger:** This spice contains natural anti-inflammatory effects and is often used as a common remedy for inflammation-related conditions. Ginger may help to calm arthritis pain by lowering hormone levels that induce inflammation.

- **Flaxseed:** Flaxseeds are rich in omega-3 fatty acids, particularly in the form alpha-linolenic acid (ALA). They also are rich in fiber, antioxidants, and lignans, which contain antioxidant and plant estrogen qualities. Both ALA and lignans may help reduce inflammation by blocking the release of certain pro-inflammatory compounds.

Acid Reflux

Acid reflux occurs when the liquid content from your stomach, or gastric acid, backs up (refluxes) into the esophagus through the lower esophageal sphincter (LES) muscle, hence the term "acid reflux." This acid causes irritation of the lining of the esophagus, resulting in heartburn. When this problem becomes chronic, it's known as gastroesophageal reflux disease (GERD).

Food can be a major culprit in acid reflux. Not everyone responds to the same foods in the same ways. If you suffer with acid reflux and/or GERD, it's important to pinpoint the foods that individually trigger your symptoms so you can avoid them. Although it's not a one-food-fits-all situation, there are some foods that in general can aggravate acid reflux symptoms and some that may just help.

Hazard foods that can trigger acid reflux include:

- **High-fat foods:** These types of foods may not be high in acidity and get as much press when it comes to heartburn, but they can take a toll on GERD sufferers. Higher-fat foods take more time and stomach acid to digest, which delays stomach emptying and can relax the LES. This, in turn, allows for your stomach to increase acid production as well as become bloated, both of which will worsen acid reflux symptoms.

- **Carbonated beverages:** Those tiny little bubbles from carbonation that seem so harmless in our favorite soft drink can often trigger acid reflux symptoms. The bubbles expand inside the stomach, which in turn increases pressure on the esophageal sphincter, promoting symptoms of reflux such as heartburn. In addition, because the carbonation increases stomach pressure, it tends to cause burping, which can cause the LES to open, again increasing your chances of acid reflux. Soft drinks that are both carbonated and contain caffeine are even worse.

- **Citrus fruits and tomato products:** As healthy as these fruits and veggies are, they tend to commonly cause or worsen acid reflux symptoms. The NIH has identified citrus fruits such as oranges, lemons, limes, and grapefruit along with tomatoes and tomato-based products as major offenders of acid reflux. These foods are highly acidic and likely to cause heartburn in those who are prone to it, especially if consumed on an empty stomach. Other vegetables such as broccoli, cauliflower, cabbage, and brussels sprouts can be gassy and therefore cause acid reflux symptoms, so experiment to see what you can tolerate.

- **Chocolate:** This tasty food is a favorite for many, but unfortunately for some, chocolate can be a common trigger for heartburn. Chocolate contains a chemical called methylxanthine that can relax the LES, allowing acid to flow back up into the esophagus. Chocolate also contains caffeine and other stimulants such as theobromine, is higher in fat, and contains cocoa, all of which can agitate reflux. Although health-wise dark chocolate is better for us, it's still chocolate and not great for those who suffer with acid reflux.

Solution foods that can help prevent acid reflux include:

- **Almonds:** Not only are they healthy, but if you're a nut lover you'll be happy to know that almonds, whether roasted, salted, or unsalted, can be effective in treating heartburn symptoms for some people. Almonds are an alkaline-producing food and can help balance the pH in your GI tract, lowering the acid and helping to reduce heartburn. Try popping three or four almonds right after a meal or snack, chewing them up well so that the oil is released from the nut. Almonds are a good source of calcium and "healthy" fats, but keep in mind that they're also high in calories, so stick to just a few. Although high in "good" fats, they also can cause heartburn in some—especially if eaten in large amounts.

- **Low-fat yogurt:** This yogurt can be beneficial for acid reflux due to the probiotics they contain. Probiotics are "friendly" bacteria that are present in and essential for a healthy digestive system. Yogurt is one of the best ways to consume probiotics, as it contains live strains of these good bacteria. Eating yogurt with probiotics can help restore and maintain the natural pH balance of the gut, which can help reduce the effects of acid reflux. Opt for Greek yogurt, which is higher in protein, and always double-check that the label states, "Live and active cultures."

- **Oatmeal:** Start your day with oatmeal instead of a greasy pork-filled breakfast, which can and probably will trigger acid reflux symptoms. Oatmeal is low in fat and high in fiber and can soothe your stomach. Including other higher-fiber foods in your daily diet can help naturally lessen your chances of experiencing acid reflux.

- **Bananas:** This healthy fruit can have an antacid effect on your stomach as well as remove a particular type of bacteria linked to ulcer formation. In addition, bananas have a naturally low acid content. Try a bite of banana shortly before a meal, with a meal, or shortly afterward to see if it brings any relief. Eat a banana anytime during the day you feel heartburn, or add them to cereal, oatmeal, yogurt, smoothies, etc. Eat bananas at the right time; if they're under-ripe they have a higher acid content, so make sure they're ripened and not too green on the outside.

Lifestyle

Not only are you what you eat, but you are what you do as well. Your lifestyle in general, besides your diet, can greatly affect many aspects of your health. Smart eating goes hand-in-hand with other lifestyle habits, including exercise, sleep, and de-stressing.

Exercise

Exercise is a habit that plays an extremely important role in managing your weight and your overall health. Everyone should exercise as part of a healthy lifestyle. Exercise doesn't have to mean hours at the gym. It means simply taking part in anything that helps to get your body moving. The goal is to get active and stay active on a regular basis, along with maintaining a healthy diet plan.

In addition, being more active in your everyday routines can be helpful. Forget about all the modern conveniences we have these days and take stairs instead of elevators, walk into the bank instead of using the drive-thru, and get off the electronic devices and walk the dog, wash the car, or work in the yard.

If you're not sure why you should exercise regularly, here are just a few of its many benefits:

- Manages blood sugar levels.

- Maintains and/or reduces body weight.

- Keeps your heart healthy by lowering both your resting heart rate and your blood pressure.

- Helps to lower "bad" cholesterol (LDL) and increase "good" cholesterol (HDL), as well as lower triglyceride levels.

- Increases blood circulation, especially to your extremities.

- Reduces the physical and mental implications of stress and depression.

- Increases your energy levels.

- Helps you to sleep better.

- Improves balance and joint flexibility.

- Helps you feel better overall, both physically and mentally.

- Decreases your risk for many chronic illnesses.

NOTABLE INSIGHT

For healthy adults, the HHS recommends getting at least 150 minutes of moderate aerobic activity or 75 minutes of vigorous activity weekly. They also recommend strength training at least twice weekly.

Starting an exercise regimen doesn't need to be difficult. It can be as easy as walking or as involved as joining a gym. Whatever you decide to do, make sure you do it consistently and you engage in activities that challenge your body. Always check with your doctor first before starting an exercise plan.

Sleep

Not getting enough sleep won't only make you feel tired, it can also contribute to health issues. Most people should get between 7 and 9 hours of sleep each night. But with our busy schedules there never seems to be enough hours in the day, so we steal hours from our sleep time.

You may not even realize it but not getting enough of those ZZZZs at night can lead to serious issues, including:

- Overweight and obesity
- Heart disease
- Type 2 diabetes
- Chronic headaches
- Depression
- Difficulty concentrating
- Fatigue

Not taking the initiative to go to bed earlier and get a good night's sleep can be different than not being able to sleep and/or having a type of sleep disorder. If you have problems sleeping, try some easy solutions on your own such as a darkened room, relaxing before bed, no caffeine after a certain time, exercise, turning your electronics off an hour before bedtime, and so on. If nothing seems to work for you, it's important enough to your overall health to see your doctor and work out a plan.

De-Stress

Stress is something we all deal with at one time or another. But for some, it becomes an everyday occurrence and can begin to affect overall health. Stress can begin to make you feel fatigued, depressed, irritable, uptight, and unable to concentrate. Chronic stress can be detrimental to your health, contributing to everything from daily headaches to obesity, heart disease, Alzheimer's disease, type 2 diabetes, acid reflux, stomach issues, anxiety, and even asthma.

Utilizing different relaxation therapies to calm stress and anxiety can help put you on the road to better health. Whether these stress-management therapies are for you or not is up to you and your doctor.

Stress-management therapies may include:

- A relaxing type of yoga
- Acupuncture
- Reiki
- Massage
- Exercise
- Guided imagery
- Deep-breathing techniques

If necessary, speak to your doctor and get help.

Genetics

Most of what we've discussed in this chapter are issues we have control of in our life. However, there is one issue we don't have control over when it comes to our health, and that's our family genes. When we come into this world, we inherit a complete set of genes from both of our parents. These genes can greatly influence and predict our health and our risk for chronic diseases, especially heart disease, cancer, diabetes, autoimmune disorders, and psychological disorders. Therefore, it's vital to know your family health history. This doesn't mean you'll absolutely be passed down a health issue or two, but it does mean you may need to be more vigilant when it comes to your healthy overall lifestyle to prevent or manage them, and get regular checkups with your doctor.

The Least You Need to Know

- We need to feed our bodies with the right type of fuel on a regular basis in order to feel our best and reduce the risk of chronic disease.

- Although certain foods are unhealthy and others act as part of the solution to common health issues, there's no single food that can cause them all or fix them all. It's about the synergy of food and eating a healthy daily diet that makes the difference.

- How we physically treat our body can determine our risk for both common health issues and chronic disease.

- We do have control over what we eat and how we treat our body. We can make positive changes and implement them long term with some effort, self-discipline, and determination.

- One determinant we can't control is our family history and genes. However, knowing our family history can be a motivator for making necessary lifestyle changes in order to prevent or manage health problems.

The Mind/Body Connection

The food we eat nourishes the body, mind, and soul. It supports us with vital nutrients we can't live without, provides a feeling of comfort, and reconnects us emotionally to a place in time when we enjoyed eating particular dishes. Unfortunately, our relationship with food can become a mental tug of war where we become vulnerable to the little voices in our head. We may unknowingly contribute to the problem by causing our bodies to crave certain foods and act impulsively about what we eat or don't eat. The lack or abundance of certain foods and nutrients as shown in recent research leads to health conditions and diseases such as obesity, depression, and Alzheimer's disease.

Achieving optimum health through food is possible. We can use food to affect our mood and mental state and to prevent disease. Changing our diet and our relationship with food can help us feel better and live a longer healthier life.

In This Chapter

- How the mind communicates with the body about food
- Food and its impact on your mental state
- The role of a healthy diet in disease prevention
- Current research and what it reveals about the mind/body connection

Mind Control

Our brain can work for or against us when it comes to eating. By listening to our body's cues, food can help us achieve an optimal body environment where it helps us think more clearly and have more energy. It seems everyone would want to line up to get more of this. On the other hand, if our schedules and lifestyle have become so hectic that we put our self-care last, most likely we have altered our natural relationship with food. This alteration can cause serious health issues and put us on the road to disease.

Mindless Eating

As a young child you intuitively knew when you were hungry and quickly alerted your parents by crying loudly. Liquid nourishment was immediately provided and you ate until you were full. It's a simple concept that unfortunately many Americans can no longer follow. There are numerous reasons we tell ourselves why we've altered our natural state. These reasons range from busy schedules to family commitments, jobs, travel, etc. This has led to undereating, overeating, and a general feeling of "dis-ease."

How can we expect ultimate performance and longevity from our body when we treat it so poorly? Think of your hunger cues as your body's doorbell. If someone rings your doorbell, the correct response would be to answer it. When your brain fuel is running low, your brain sends out a message and your stomach grumbles. Many times we ignore the body's doorbell. This leads to a lack of nutrients for our brain because we're overhungry, setting us up for overeating at the next meal. The next thing you know, you've consumed too much food and put yourself into a "food coma." Your body is now working overtime trying to utilize this large food payload. Your brain is foggy and makes you feel worse than you did before you ate.

By following this practice, you've taught your body it may be a long time before your next meal. Your brain sends out a hunger message in order to "stockpile" food. It believes food must be scarce since you're unable to feed it on a regular schedule and are ignoring the doorbell. How do you change this behavior and get back on the track to good eating habits? By eating intuitively.

Intuitive Eating

Intuitive eating is being mindful of what your body is telling you. It involves listening to your body's cues about hunger, *satiety,* emotional state, and taste. It helps to identify and eliminate the good food/bad food rhetoric in our minds and teaches us to make positive changes.

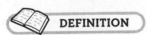 **DEFINITION**

Satiety is the feeling of fullness after eating. It takes about 20 minutes for your brain to receive the message of fullness after consumption of a meal.

The three core principles of intuitive eating are unrestricted eating based on need, following hunger cues as opposed to eating for emotional reasons, and relying on your internal signals for fullness and satiety. This practice is also referred to as mindful eating.

Intuitive or mindful eating practices not being judgmental toward your emotions and physical feelings. It also removes outside influences such as marketing. Oftentimes the practice of being mindful involves some form of meditation. This practice has shown to decrease stress and depression. A 2009 study showed a high body image score in individuals practicing mindfulness through yoga, meditation, and intuitive eating.

The Academy of Nutrition and Dietetics (AND) states that intuitive eating interventions have been shown to decrease negative eating behaviors as well as symptoms of anxiety and depression. Practicing mindful eating fosters increased self-esteem, along with a healthier body image and relationship with food.

Psychological flexibility is used in fostering intuitive eating. Individuals with increased levels of psychological flexibility give themselves unconditional permission to eat for physical reasons. Individuals who practice these concepts generally have a lower BMI and better acceptance of their feelings in regard to their weight, and in turn, practice more intuitive eating approaches.

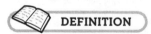 **DEFINITION**

> **Psychological flexibility** involves keeping your long-term goals and values in sight. Present emotions and behaviors don't always fall in line with your overall values. Impulsive behavior and disruptive thoughts can undermine what you really want. Being able to adapt to various situations without losing sight of your goals is crucial for your well-being. Psychological flexibility is measured using a scale called the Acceptance and Action Questionnaire (AAQ). In several studies, a low AAQ indicates increased anxiety, reduced work performance, and lowered quality of life.

Gut Microbes

The tiny bacteria living in the gut is beneficial for breaking down fiber and creating a variety of vitamins. However, these microbes are also living organisms and are not doing this out of the kindness of their heart. The goal of the bacteria is to thrive and reproduce. They require certain nutrients to do so.

A review published in *BioEssays* states that gut bacteria have the ability to increase intake of foods the body needs to survive and thrive. By creating cravings for particular foods through the vagus nerve, our brain gets the message from our gut to eat. If their needs are not met, the bacteria have the ability to create a state of dissatisfaction in our gut, likely leading to discomfort or pain.

Depending on the strains of bacteria, the brain receives messages to increase intake of certain types of foods. Some bacteria thrive on carbohydrates. Other strains need polysaccharides (sugars) or fat components to survive. Sending too many calories to the gut bacteria may also increase specific strains and upset the balance of microbes in your gut.

Making changes in our diet and consuming foods such as pre- and probiotics can help control our gut bacteria and the messages they're sending to our brain. By eating a balanced diet with an optimal amount of energy, we can rewire the bacteria to survive on new foods.

Food and Mood

What you eat or don't eat will affect your brain chemistry. There are a host of hormones and chemicals that help regulate your body and participate in the communication process with your self. For example, if you're craving carbohydrates, it may be that your blood sugar levels have dropped and you need more glucose for the brain to run efficiently. As glycogen (the storage form of glucose) drops, your blood sugar drops. Next, your brain sends out a message to release a nerve chemical, which stimulates appetite and causes you to crave carbohydrates.

After consumption of those delicious carbs, the chemical levels in your body return to normal along with blood sugar levels.

Stress is also an instigator in craving carbohydrates, and it puts your food cravings into high gear. When you're extremely stressed, your adrenal glands release a hormone that activates a brain chemical and stimulates the desire for carbohydrates. They decrease your stress level by helping to soothe and calm you. Repeating this cycle due to stress can lead to unwanted weight gain.

A study published in *The British Journal of Nutrition* showed improvements in mood when individuals followed a diet low in sodium and high in potassium. During the study, individuals on low-sodium diets had lower urinary excretion and exhibited fewer symptoms of anger and vigor. Those who had a higher dietary intakes of potassium and magnesium also had higher urinary excretion levels of potassium and magnesium along with reduced symptoms of fatigue and vigor, as well as increased *cortisol* levels. The study points out the connection between low sodium to potassium ratio and reduced feelings of anger and overall depression. Participants on the prescribed low-sodium, high-potassium diet also had an improved global mood score over those on the diet replicating the Dietary Approaches to Stop Hypertension (DASH) diet.

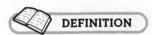 **DEFINITION**

> **Cortisol** is a hormone thought to play a role in the stress response. Reduced levels of cortisol are found in individuals with depression and type 2 diabetes.

How we feel about our food choices influences our mood. A study published in *Appetite* states a link between perceived ingestion of calories and mood. Participants were given one of two breakfasts, one cereal and one a muffin, which were identical in calories and nutrient make-up. Participants believed the breakfast of cereal was lower in calories, and those individuals who ate the cereal reported higher body image, mood, and satiety.

Food Frenzy

Oftentimes it seems that eating food is a real chore. What to eat? When to eat? How much to eat? These are all very good questions. It may be so overwhelming that you decide to eat whatever is the fastest and easiest thing to grab. This causes a cascade of detrimental effects that can keep your body in a vicious cycle of feeling lousy, with low energy and a foggy brain state. It's like you have a cold and can't think clearly. Sometimes we think it's related to our age or health status, which can be partially true. What it really comes down to is providing your body the nutrients it needs to function at its very best.

Eating on a regular schedule has been shown to affect mood. In a study published in *Appetite*, individuals in a cafeteria setting were surveyed about their mood during the morning. The participants, both male and female, who reported they ate breakfast also reported a better mood and more relaxed feeling throughout the morning.

The energy composition of meals may be as important as the timing. A study in *Physiology & Behavior* showed a link between fat content at breakfast and mood. Individuals eating a high-fat breakfast showed more signs of lethargy, decreased attentiveness, and depressed feelings. The same link was not seen at lunch.

All Systems Go

When you eat a healthy diet throughout the day, your body works more efficiently. Your mood is better, and you have more energy and stamina. It prevents those highs and lows of blood sugar along with preventing the release of a host of hormone- and appetite-stimulating chemicals that drive us to eat. Eating well helps us think more clearly, especially about the food choices we make. Food has an important role in our lives, and eating the right foods can make a positive impact on our health and longevity.

The Sleep Connection

The National Sleep Foundation reports a decrease of two hours of sleep per day for the average American over the last century. Yet sleep is critical for mood, work performance, and good health. Not everyone gets a good night's sleep. About 40 percent of Americans spend a few nights a week tossing and turning. Those with chronic pain face a sleep debt of close to 45 minutes every night. Stress and poor health appear to contribute to inadequate sleep patterns.

The obesity epidemic may also be partly caused by poor sleep. The body's hormones help control its many functions. The hormones leptin and grehlin affect hunger, satiety, and weight loss and gain. Sleep, or the lack thereof, has been shown to significantly affect these and other hormone levels.

Sleep and Hormones

Grehlin is a hormone found in the GI tract that is released when there's an inadequate supply of energy. This hormone stimulates the satiety center in the brain, called the hypothalamus, and tells you to eat. Think of "ghrelin gain."

Leptin is a hormone released by the adipocytes (fat cells) to help you lose weight. When leptin levels rise, the body burns fat. Leptin levels are directly affected by caloric intake. Think "leptin lose."

In addition to calories, sleep has the ability to increase circulating leptin levels. According to researchers at the University of Chicago, cortisol and insulin have been shown to work together to control leptin levels.

Studies have shown that individuals with high BMI generally have low levels of ghrelin and high levels of leptin. One theory is that the constant release of leptin during overeating suppresses levels of ghrelin.

In a research study looking at sleep and leptin levels, participants were assigned sleep times of 4-, 8-, and 12-hour spans. The participants' leptin levels changed significantly based on sleep time allowed, even when their weight stayed stable. During the study, individuals on the 12-hour sleep plan had significantly higher leptin levels above the 4-hour sleep patterns.

The Wisconsin Sleep Cohort Study found healthy adults experienced a drop in leptin and an increase in ghrelin in conjunction with self-reported deficiency in sleep. The Research Network on Mind-Body Interactions of the MacArthur Foundation reports individuals who had only 4 hours sleep for two consecutive nights already experienced a drop in leptin and an increase in ghrelin.

It's thought the decreased leptin levels during reduced sleep help account for the increased time awake, and thus the increased caloric need to fuel the body. Increased cortisol levels are negatively correlated with leptin levels. When cortisol was high (during stress), leptin levels decreased. Glucocorticoids, such as cortisol, are known to increase hunger and food consumption.

Researchers believe hunger and eating patterns may be stimulated by lack of sleep earlier in the day.

Diet in Shift Workers

Approximately 20 percent of workers in America work shifts that include all or a portion of the night hours. These workers have a propensity for less than healthy habits and a higher risk for specific health conditions like heart disease, diabetes, mood and digestive disorders along with hormonal imbalance. Shift workers experience a change in the quantity and quality of food intake in addition to a higher risk for home life and personal and social problems.

In a study comparing shift and day workers' dietary intake, researchers at Université Toulouse III found shift workers consumed more meals than their counterparts working the day shift. The energy intake between the groups was comparable, but the quantity and quality varied. Shift workers ate almost one third less at breakfast than their counterparts, and a slightly smaller lunch. The subsequent meals made up for the previous smaller meals with an increase in fat and saturated fat over the daytime workers.

A review article in the *International Journal of Endocrinology* reported nighttime shift workers consumed over half of their calories in the evening and at night. Nighttime feeding also accounted for an additional 350 to 500 calories a day. Eating at times when the *circadian rhythm* is low increases insulin resistance and is biologically less effective than feeding during daytime hours.

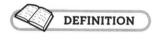

DEFINITION

The natural clock inside your body controlling hormone levels and sleep-wake cycles is called the **circadian rhythm** or cycle. This natural rhythm closely follows a 24-hour clock. It's stimulated by environmental factors such as availability of light and dark. The circadian clock stimulates eating and sleeping patterns and is affected by lack or inconsistent amounts of sleep.

Connection Between Food and Mood Disorders

There are numerous human studies involving men, women, and children supporting the relationship between a healthy diet and a decreased risk of disease. A diet high in macro- and micronutrients is positively correlated with an improved mental state, greater energy, and delayed onset of certain conditions and diseases such as depression, dementia, and Alzheimer's. Researchers found that certain foods and nutrients can have a beneficial effect on the quality of life and longevity.

The Canadian Journal of Psychiatry published a study showing the effects of low zinc levels on increased mania and depression. Individuals functioning at a higher psychological level had an increased intake of calcium, magnesium, phosphorous, potassium, iron, and zinc. This intake could be from both food and supplements.

Seasonal Affective Disorder (SAD)

Changes due to circadian rhythm affect approximately 5 percent of Americans. Seasonal affective disorder (SAD) is characterized by disturbances in mood patterns with seasonal variations. Symptoms generally worsen in the darker winter months and lessen in the summer months. Symptoms include food cravings, increased appetite, carbohydrate intake, weight gain, fatigue, and increased sleep.

NOTABLE INSIGHT

The "winter blues" is also called seasonal affective disorder. The condition generally begins in your 20s, but the risk of acquiring it increases as you age. Some individuals may gain upwards of 20 pounds and sleep an additional four hours a night. Individuals in parts of the world where there are more hours of night than day during the winter months are at a higher risk of having the disorder.

Research published in *Chronobiology* reports individuals afflicted with SAD crave an increased level of carbohydrates in the evening hours. This ingestion of higher levels of carbohydrates by SAD sufferers seems to decrease their level of depression and increase their energy. It appears glucose increases the reaction of the retina to light.

Depression

Depression is one of the most common mental disorders worldwide—it's estimated that 350 million people are affected. Depression can be mild, moderate, or severe. Depression is a persistent sadness with feelings of hopelessness and loss of interest in life, especially with activities that used to bring pleasure. There are many different types of depression. They include major depression, persistent depressive disorder, psychotic depression, postpartum depression, seasonal affective disorder, and bipolar disorder. Treatment typically involves medication and psychotherapy.

Studies have shown a relationship between depression and health. A research study published in *The Journal of the American Board of Family Medicine* reported there was a connection between having a very low magnesium intake and an increased incidence of depression. This was especially pertinent in younger adults.

Magnesium is found in most vegetables and fruits. It's recommended Americans consume 2,400 milligrams of magnesium every day.

Another researcher examined the impact of a high-protein diet and severely depressed moods. They found the high-protein diet offered protection from depression in men but adversely affected women. Researchers believe the difference is due to the way the body metabolizes energy and the chemical effect on the brain.

There were also apparent differences in baseline nutrient values between men and women.

An additional study found a link between an increase in depressive symptoms in mid- and late-life adults. Women with high cholesterol levels had more rapid onset of depressive symptoms and interpersonal problems. The same increase was not seen in men.

Cognitive Decline

Nutrition plays a key role in reducing and delaying the symptoms associated with cognitive decline. Healthy eating patterns rather than individual foods have been shown to have the largest impact. The nutrients in diets, such as the Mediterranean diet, work together in a synergetic manner. These patterns have been reported to work for cognitive decline, dementia, and Alzheimer's disease.

Alzheimer's disease is the most common type of dementia. In 2015, it was estimated that there were 5.3 million Americans suffering from this disease. Alzheimer's causes a decline in memory and thinking abilities. It renders people unable to communicate and/or perform daily activities of living. A recent study in the *American Society for Nutrition* reviewed dietary patterns, cognitive decline, and dementia. It found less cognitive decline, dementia, and Alzheimer's disease among people who follow a Mediterranean diet.

 NOTABLE INSIGHT

The DASH diet was developed to help people reduce blood pressure by consuming foods high in potassium, calcium, and magnesium, and low in sodium. The diet focuses on whole grains, vegetables, fruits, low-fat dairy, and lean proteins along with nuts, seeds, and legumes.

Another study looked at the differences between the Mediterranean diet, the DASH diet, and a hybrid of the Mediterranean and the DASH called the MIND diet.

Researchers found that while all three diets helped reduce the risk of Alzheimer's, those who strictly followed the MIND diet were able to reduce their risk by 53 percent and those who only moderately followed the diet by 35 percent. These are impressive findings showing that many people could markedly improve their health through food.

The MIND diet differs from the other two diets by specifically recommending the intake of berries and green leafy vegetables, and makes no recommendations for high fruit, dairy, and potato intake. It also reduces the total servings of fish to once per week.

Serotonin Sensitive Disorders

Serotonin is a *neurotransmitter* that contributes to feelings of wellbeing and happiness. Vitamin D and omega-3 fatty acids are involved in production and activation of serotonin. A research article published recently suggests supplementation of these nutrients could help treat symptoms of attention deficit hyperactivity disorder (ADHD), bipolar disorder, schizophrenia, impulsive behavior, and obsessive-compulsive disorder (OCD). This type of supplementation would have fewer side effects than traditional medications currently used to treat these issues. Researchers mentioned it's common for people with these types of conditions to be deficient in many nutrients. Additionally, they stressed the importance of adequate vitamin B_6 and iron due to its role in serotonin synthesis.

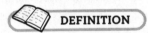 **DEFINITION**

Neurotransmitters are chemicals responsible for sending communication signals throughout your body. They can either stimulate the brain or calm the brain. Stress, poor diet, genetics, drugs, alcohol, and caffeine adversely affect neurotransmitter levels.

The Least You Need to Know

- A healthy diet can lead to mental clarity.
- What you eat affects your mind/body connection.
- Always listen to your body's hunger and satiety signals.
- Key nutrients can help prevent or delay the onset of certain diseases and conditions.

The Basics of Nutrition

The human body is amazing in its ability to absorb and digest nutrients from the foods you eat. In this part, we cover the fundamentals of digestion and explain how your body uses nutrients like carbohydrates, proteins, and fats, along with vitamins and minerals to support good health. We'll teach you how much of each nutrient you need and show you where to obtain it. We'll also look at what happens when the digestive process goes awry and leads to disease. You'll learn how to recognize the signs and symptoms and what you can do about it.

In addition, we'll also explain the differences between simple and complex carbs and look at the role of fiber in your diet. We'll also review the differences between plant-based and animal-based proteins, and how they affect your health. Finally, we'll look at the role of fats—the good ones and the ones to avoid, and discuss what you need to know in terms of vitamins, minerals, and phytonutrients..

Digestion 101

The digestive process receives impulses from your five senses: sight, smell, taste, auditory, and touch. When you walk into a bakery, the sight and smell of freshly baked pastries is enough to get your digestive juices flowing. The digestion and absorption of food is a step-by-step process that involves a host of actions from various organs and metabolic processes.

In this chapter, we'll look at how the nutrients in foods are utilized by your body for growth, repair, and protection. We'll explore what occurs throughout each step in the digestive tract, along with the intricate processes of converting food into usable components. Additionally, we'll examine what happens when a problem in the digestive process occurs and learn the best ways to deal with the issue.

In This Chapter

- The steps of the digestion process
- How your body absorbs nutrients from food
- When food can physically hurt?
- How to strengthen your gut with pro- and prebiotics
- Why does your body need water?

Where Does It Begin?

The journey through the digestive system physically begins in the mouth. Food travels through the oral cavity, esophagus, and stomach, which are referred to as your upper digestive tract. The lower digestive tract includes the small and large intestines, with assistance from organs like the pancreas, liver, and gallbladder, which aid in the release of enzymes and chemicals into the intestines to help break down the nutrients. Through this chemical and mechanical action, food is broken down into small molecules your body can readily absorb.

The Mouth

The first step of digestion occurs in the mouth. The function of the mouth is to mechanically break down foods through the action of chewing, which grinds the foods into smaller particles to maximize access to nutrients. Strong jaw muscles also provide power to assist in this step. As food is broken down, saliva produced by the salivary glands adds moisture. Saliva is made up of 99.5 percent water, along with enzymes and mucus. There are three types of salivary glands: parotid, sublingual, and submandibular, which are located in the oral cavity above and below your teeth.

Amylase is the first enzyme contained in your saliva that acts on the food in its moistened state, which begins breaking down the bonds that hold starch molecules together. The tongue and back of the mouth also contain glands that secrete lingual lipase, another enzyme that acts on fats like triglycerides upon their arrival in the stomach. The enzyme's role is minimal, and these particular enzymatic actions are more prevalent in infants to aid in the digestion of milk fats. This enzyme's release decreases with age.

The action of swallowing is a voluntary muscle action initiated by you. However, it's the brain that regulates the remaining involuntary swallowing processes that take place. Food must first pass through the pharynx, which is basically a 5-inch section in the back of the throat beginning at the base of the skull with openings to the nasal passageways and trachea, also known as the windpipe.

As food passes down the back of the throat, the larynx, which is part of the respiratory system and houses your vocal cords, receives a signal. The larynx moves up, which allows the epiglottis (a flap of skin) to slide over and cover the trachea to prevent food from going down into your windpipe and choking you. The larynx is made up of cartilage and is visibly recognizable on the outside front of the neck. It's commonly referred to as the Adam's apple.

NOTABLE INSIGHT

Close to 3,000 adults die every year due to choking, which occurs when the trachea or windpipe, which leads to the lungs, becomes blocked. In most cases, it's blocked by food. The Heimlich maneuver can be performed to remove the food, by grasping the choking person around the waist from behind with hands clasped and giving a short thrust in an upward motion directly below the diaphragm. This motion expels air from the lungs and hopefully dislodges the food from the blocked airway.

The swallowed food is referred to as a "bolus." Once the bolus passes through the pharynx, it moves into the esophagus. The esophagus is a hollow tube about 10 inches in length and 1 inch in diameter. It runs from the base of the pharynx to the stomach, and its only function is to transport food. The presence of the food stimulates the parasympathetic nerves, which are responsible for propelling the food down into the stomach. This involuntary muscle action is called *peristalsis*. Peristalsis is the alternating of involuntary muscle contractions and relaxations to cause a wave-like movement. At the end of the esophagus is the lower esophageal *sphincter,* which controls the flow of food into the stomach.

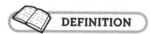

DEFINITION

A **sphincter** is a circular muscle portal between key passages in the GI tract that controls the release of food.

The Stomach

The lower esophageal sphincter controls entry of the bolus into the stomach. As you swallow food, the sphincter relaxes due to an overall drop in pressure. Neural and hormonal regulators manage pressure levels within the sphincter. Once relaxed, the sphincter allows the food to pass into the stomach. The volume of an adult stomach when empty is equivalent to about $1/4$ cup. It can expand to hold 4 to 6 cups or even more—think of all those food-eating contests. Food remains in your stomach for 2 to 6 hours where it's chemically and mechanically broken down into small molecules your body can readily absorb.

The stomach is located on the left side of your body under your diaphragm at the base of your lungs. It has three types of muscles: longitudinal, circular, and diagonal. Their function is to help expand and contract to aid in combining food with the acidic contents of the stomach.

The stomach consists of four main parts: the *cardia, fundus, body,* and *antrum.* The antrum, the lower third of the stomach, is where most of the action takes place. The cardia is the top portion of the stomach near where food enters. The section to the right of the cardia is the fundus. The central part of the stomach is where food is held. The stomach is lined in folds called *rugae.* These folds can flatten out and allow the stomach to expand and accommodate a large amount of food.

The antrum is responsible for using the muscles to churn and mix up all that food with the gastric juices and enzymes contained in the stomach.

The stomach is protected from its acidic contents by a thick mucous membrane. Just below the mucous lining are epithelial cells that contain gastric glands and release a variety of digestive juices. What's released is dependent on their particular location within the stomach. The glands secrete hydrochloric acid (HCL), mucus, water, electrolytes, *intrinsic factor,* and enzymes. Gastric juices are very acidic, with a pH around 2 in comparison to battery acid at 0.

The primary function of HCL is to activate pepsin, the enzyme needed to help break apart bonds within proteins, kill incoming foreign bacteria from foods you eat, and aid in the release of nutrients. After the food has been worked over by the stomach actions, it resembles a thin watery pastelike substance called *chyme.* Chyme will exit the stomach about a teaspoon at a time through the pyloric sphincter and into the small intestine.

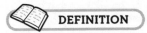 **DEFINITION**

> **Intrinsic factor** is a protein produced by cells in the stomach wall. It is required for the absorption of vitamin B_{12}. **Chyme** is partially digested semifluid mass of food found in the stomach that passes from the stomach into the small intestine.

The Small Intestine

The small intestine is the primary site of nutrient digestion and absorption. It's approximately 21 feet in length and about 1 inch in diameter. The longitudinal and circular muscles that make up the length of the tube are designed to help propel the food through the intestines via wavelike motions.

The small intestine is composed of three sections: the *duodenum, jejunum,* and *ileum.* The intestine, like the stomach, is covered in a thick layer of mucus to protect it from the highly acidic environment. Once the chyme from the stomach enters the first section of the intestine, called the duodenum, specialized cells residing in the lining begin to release alkaline secretions to help neutralize the acidic chyme. It then receives a dose of secretions from the pancreas, which contains bicarbonate to ensure the acid has been neutralized. If by chance there is an error in the levels of pH and the acid is not neutralized, then erosion will occur in the lining over time and cause the development of an ulcer.

The pancreatic enzymes digest approximately half of all carbohydrates and proteins and almost all of the fat. Bile is excreted from the gallbladder where it travels through a duct into the duodenum. Bile is made by the liver and stored in the gallbladder. It consists of acids, salts, cholesterol, phospholipids, and bile pigments. Bile's role in the digestive process is to emulsify fats. Specifically, it connects water and fat molecules together in order to allow the enzymes to access and digest them.

The lining of the intestines contains circular mucosal folds, which look like steep, rolling hills with very deep valleys. The purpose of these folds is to increase the surface area to maximize nutrient absorption. Each of the folds is also covered in a layer of fingerlike projections called *villi*. These villi are wrapped in epithelial cells. Just beneath those cells are blood capillaries and lymph vessels ready to absorb and transport the nutrients throughout the body.

Additionally, the villi are covered in microvilli, which are referred to as the "brush border." Microvilli are hairlike projections that contain digestive enzymes from the mucosa cells in the lining. These enzymes break up partially digested carbohydrates and proteins, allowing the nutrients to be readily absorbed into the brush-border cells where they can then move into the blood or lymph fluids.

 NOTABLE INSIGHT

Your small intestine has the largest surface area in your body. Picture the size of a tennis court (78 feet long × 36 feet wide). That's about the same amount of square footage you have available for your body to absorb nutrients from the food you eat.

The majority of the absorption of digested nutrients occurs in the upper portion of the small intestine. Carbohydrates, proteins, fats, vitamins, and minerals are absorbed in each distinct section of the duodenum, jejunum, and ileum. The mechanism of absorption of the nutrients is generally through one of four ways:

1. Diffusion: Nutrients pass directly into the next membrane.

2. Facilitated diffusion: Nutrients need a carrier to assist in passing through the membrane wall.

3. Active transport: Molecules need a little extra boost of energy from adenosine triphosphate (ATP) to pass through the membrane wall.

4. Pinocytosis: Nutrients are surrounded by the membrane and then pinched off and absorbed into the membrane.

Leftovers that cannot be absorbed, such as fiber, dead cells, salt, bile, and water, are passed on to the large intestine.

The Large Intestine (Colon)

Chyme is passed from the small intestine to the large intestine through the ileocecal valve into the large intestine. The length of the intestine is 5 feet long and about 3 inches in diameter. The beginning of your large intestine is called the *cecum*. The colon, which we commonly refer to as the large intestine, is made up of the *ascending colon, transverse colon, descending colon,* and *sigmoid colon.* The overall muscle structure differs from the small intestine, as it is designed to allow for indentions that, when filled with chyme, bulge outward. This increases the length of time the chyme has to be in contact within the intestinal wall, allowing for optimal absorption of nutrients. Chyme can remain in the colon for 1 to 3 days. During that time, sodium, potassium, chloride, vitamin K, biotin, and water are absorbed. What remains is mostly fiber.

The large intestine contains its own world of microflora or bacteria. The bacteria use the food leftovers, such as fiber, to help produce some vitamins. These microorganisms also help break down and ferment this fiber. This is a crucial role of the gut flora because humans lack the enzyme to break down fiber. Once everything has been absorbed that can be, the leftover residue is propelled to the end of the colon where the rectum is located. Waste remains there until it is time to be excreted.

When Digestion Goes Wrong

Most of the time our digestive process works flawlessly. Every now and then problems occur, like an upset stomach, which can be easily remedied by over-the-counter medications. Problems can also be more serious in nature, as in the case of *ulcers,* irritable bowel syndrome (IBS), food allergies, and leaky gut syndrome. Many of these causes are directly relatable to a specific error that occurs in the digestive tract and sometimes the diagnosis is not so clear-cut. Working closely with your doctor to get your digestive tract functioning again is important for good overall health.

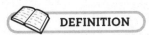 **DEFINITION**

> An **ulcer** or peptic ulcer occurs when stomach acids that digest food cause erosion in the stomach wall or duodenum. Ulcers can be caused by untreated gastroesophageal reflux disease (GERD), excessive use of aspirin and ibuprofen, or most commonly by bacterium known as *Helicobacter pylori*. While stress and spicy foods do not specifically cause ulcers, they can aggravate the symptoms.

Heartburn, Acid Reflux, and GERD

Heartburn, acid reflux, and gastroesophageal reflux disease (GERD) are often used interchangeably; however, heartburn is a symptom of acid reflux and GERD. Heartburn is literally a pain in the chest, which occurs about an hour after eating. It can be aggravated by lying down, which causes an alteration in pressure in the valve and allows seepage of the acidic chyme to backflow up into the esophagus. Many people end up in the emergency room thinking they're having a heart attack when, fortunately, it's only heartburn. The pain is caused by the acidic contents creating a burning sensation. Taking antacids can relieve it, but your doctor needs to determine the underlying cause.

Certain foods and lifestyle habits aggravate this condition by assisting in the alteration of gastric pressure or increasing the production of acid. These foods include high-fat foods, acidic foods, alcohol, nicotine, caffeine, calcium, and orange juice, along with some spices.

Typically treatment will involve eating smaller meals, which will decrease gastric pressure, and thoroughly chewing your food. It is also advised to avoid spicy or acidic foods, to drink water between meals, and to wait three hours before lying down after a meal. If you're overweight, losing just 2 percent of your body weight may help alleviate symptoms.

Acid reflux is when the stomach contents (chyme) move backwards into your esophagus. The same treatment approach for heartburn can manage the symptoms of acid reflux. However, when acid reflux is ongoing and occurs more than twice a week, it's labeled GERD and serious damage to the esophagus can occur. The acidic chyme will damage the esophageal mucosa lining and can cause inflammation and swelling. If left untreated, this inflammation and swelling can damage the esophagus by scarring and cause bleeding and ulcers. Severe damage can even progress to cancer of the esophagus.

Celiac Disease

The first known case of celiac disease dates back as far as the second century. This autoimmune disorder currently is considered to be a major public health issue on the rise. Celiac disease is four times more common today than it was 60 years ago. It affects about 1 in 100 people in the United States according to Mayo Clinic Research Education.

Celiac disease is an autoimmune disorder of the intestines and occurs when gluten, a protein found in wheat, rye, and barley, is ingested. When a person with Celiac disease consumes gluten, the protein is not broken down through the normal digestion process. It's viewed as an enemy and is attacked by the immune system. Over time, the consumption of gluten damages the small intestine, specifically villi, the small fingerlike projections that assist in nutrient absorption. Damaged villi within the intestines will lead to less nutrient absorption and potential malnutrition.

Celiac disease can occur at any age and is also considered to be hereditary. While it's not fully understood why the immune system attacks gluten and causes damage to the small intestine, it is crucial to recognize key symptoms. For children, these symptoms may include abdominal bloating and pain; chronic diarrhea; constipation; vomiting; pale, foul-smelling, or fatty stool; weight loss, fatigue; irritability and behavioral issues; and failure to thrive.

For adults, symptoms are less likely to be related to digestion. Symptoms for adults include anemia, fatigue, bone or joint pain, arthritis, depression or anxiety, tingling numbness in the hands or feet, seizures or migraines, missed menstrual periods, cankers sores in the mouth, itchy skin rash, and diarrhea.

It's important to recognize symptoms early on as this disease can lead to other serious health problems, including the development of other autoimmune disorders such as type 2 diabetes and multiple sclerosis.

The current treatment for celiac disease is a gluten-free diet, which means avoiding foods with wheat, rye, and barley. Even the smallest amount of gluten can trigger damage to the small intestine; therefore, it's important to follow a strict diet.

Inflammatory Bowel Disease (IBD)

Inflammatory bowel disease (IBD) is a general term for illnesses that result from a frequent *immune response* and chronic inflammation of the gastrointestinal (GI) tract. The two most common inflammatory bowel diseases are ulcerative colitis and Crohn's disease.

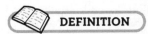 **DEFINITION**

The **immune response** is how your body recognizes and defends itself against bacteria, viruses, and substances that appear foreign and harmful.

IBD is the result of the immune system mistaking food, bacteria, and other materials that can be found in the intestines as foreign objects. The immune system triggers a response to attack the cells of the intestines. During this response, white blood cells are sent to the intestines, specifically the lining, where they cause chronic inflammation.

In Crohn's disease, inflammation affects the entire digestive tract. Only the large intestine is affected in ulcerative colitis. Both illnesses are characterized by an abnormal response to the body's immune system.

Ulcerative colitis causes sores and inflammation within the lining of the colon (large intestine) and rectum. While most cases are diagnosed before the age of 30, ulcerative colitis can affect people of any age. The cause of ulcerative colitis is unclear, although some studies show IBD results from genetic and environmental factors. When the body is exposed to antigens or foreign objects in the environment, it defends itself by producing inflammation. This reaction may be enough to "turn on" the immune system. When the immune system doesn't properly "turn off," inflammation continues to damage the body, and in this case, the large intestine. The primary goal for people with an inflammatory bowel disease is to keep their immune system healthy.

Almost half of all people with ulcerative colitis have mild symptoms. However, others may suffer from severe abdominal cramping, bloody diarrhea, nausea, and fever. The symptoms of ulcerative colitis can come and go, with fairly long periods in between flare-ups.

Complications can include bleeding from deep ulcerations, rupture of the bowel, or failure to respond to the usual medical treatments. Another complication is severe abdominal bloating. People with ulcerative colitis also have an increased risk of colon cancer. In over one fourth of patients with ulcerative colitis, medical therapy is not completely successful, and surgery may need to be considered to remove all or part of the colon (known as a colectomy). Ulcerative colitis is "cured" once the damaged colon is removed.

Unlike ulcerative colitis that affects a specific area of the GI tract, Crohn's disease is an inflammation in any location throughout the digestive tract. The majority of patients with Crohn's disease will require surgery at some point during their lives. Surgery becomes necessary in Crohn's disease when medications can no longer control the symptoms.

According to the Crohn's and Colitis Foundation of America (CCFA), as many as 700,000 Americans are affected by Crohn's disease, with both men and women being equally affected. Crohn's can appear at any age, but it's more predominant among adolescents and young adults between the ages of 15 and 35.

As with ulcerative colitis, the causes of Crohn's disease are not clearly understood. Current research shows that it can be hereditary, along with the environment contributing to the advancement of Crohn's disease.

Symptoms for Crohn's disease mimic other inflammatory bowel diseases, including abdominal cramping, bloody or fatty diarrhea, fever, and weight loss. Due to the inflamed area of the intestine, the system is unable to absorb nutrients properly. Additionally, much fluid is lost through diarrhea along with blood. As the individual has recurring flare-ups with the disease, nutrient deficiencies can develop, such as anemia.

Sometimes the GI tract can become so inflamed that it is necessary to allow it to rest. The person then must eat an liquid diet intravenously in order for the gut to have proper time to heal.

The first step in treating both ulcerative colitis and Crohn's disease is to replace lost nutrients and fluids. Diet recommendations may vary in each case, but it's important to identify food triggers in order to minimize flare-ups. Overall, a high-calorie and high-protein diet, along with a multivitamin supplement, is typically recommended. In periods of remission, high fiber is recommended to increase bowel motility.

Irritable Bowel Syndrome (IBS)

It's important to know that irritable bowel syndrome (IBS) is common and can be less severe than IBD. Doctors consider IBS a functional GI disorder. This basically means your digestive tract performs in an irregular way but without evidence of the digestive tract damage that occurs with inflammatory bowel disease.

IBS affects the large intestine and occurs when there is too much or too little movement of food within the colon. IBS is characterized by abdominal pain and discomfort along with changes in bowel movement patterns. In order to provide the right treatment to patients with IBS, doctors classify IBS into four categories based on stool consistency.

The four types of IBS are as follows:

- **IBS with constipation:** Hard or lumpy stools at least 25 percent of the time and loose or watery stools less than 25 percent of the time

- **IBS with diarrhea:** Loose or watery stools at least 25 percent of the time and hard or lumpy stools less than 25 percent of the time

- **Mixed IBS:** Hard or lumpy stools at least 25 percent of the time and loose or watery stools at least 25 percent of the time

- **Unsubtyped IBS:** Hard or lumpy stools less than 25 percent of the time and loose or watery stools less than 25 percent of the time

Physical problems such as the brain-gut signal, GI motility, bacterial infections, genetics, and food sensitivities may all contribute to the development of IBS. When the brain signals the nerves in the gut to digest food, there may be a miscommunication or abnormal response that causes IBS symptoms. These symptoms may include bloating, cramping, gas, alternating diarrhea and constipation, and mucus in the stool. IBS is also found to affect more women than men and usually occurs in people under 45 who have a family history or a mental health problem.

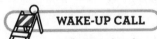 **WAKE-UP CALL**

Chronic diarrhea can lead to dehydration. A person can tolerate 3 to 4 percent loss of water but any higher than that can cause serious adverse health effects. It's important to try to replace lost fluids, especially during an illness.

Leaky Gut Syndrome

Leaky gut syndrome occurs when there's increased permeability within the intestines. This simply means that undigested food particles and toxins that would normally be blocked are able to flow into the bloodstream. These foreign particles and toxins cause the immune system to react, and often cause allergies. For example, if you eat a banana and you have leaky gut syndrome, bits of undigested banana will escape the intestines and find their way directly into the bloodstream. When this occurs, the immune system considers these particles a dangerous threat and reacts by producing antibodies and attacking healthy cells.

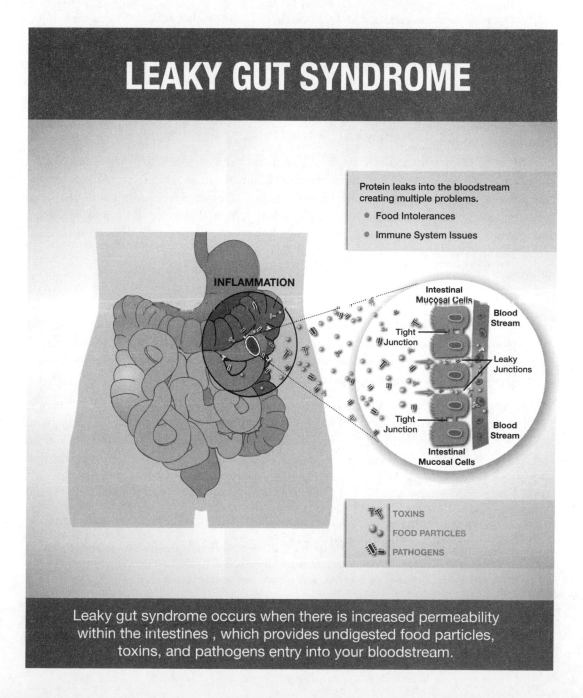

LEAKY GUT SYNDROME

Protein leaks into the bloodstream creating multiple problems.

- Food Intolerances
- Immune System Issues

INFLAMMATION

Intestinal Mucosal Cells

Blood Stream

Tight Junction

Leaky Junctions

Tight Junction

Blood Stream

Intestinal Mucosal Cells

TOXINS
FOOD PARTICLES
PATHOGENS

Leaky gut syndrome occurs when there is increased permeability within the intestines , which provides undigested food particles, toxins, and pathogens entry into your bloodstream.

There are several factors that can lead to leaky gut. One reason may be chronic constipation due to toxins in your stools. Over time, these toxins can irritate your intestinal lining, which can lead to inflammation. The constant inflammation then causes pores within the intestines to expand, leading to increased permeability in the intestinal lining.

Another possible cause of leaky gut is the imbalance of healthy gut bacteria. When there is an imbalance between the "good" and "bad" bacteria, irritation and inflammation can occur.

Establishing a diagnosis for leaky gut syndrome can be tricky, as there is a wide range of unrelated symptoms and no definitive tests to confirm. The symptoms may include gas, bloating, diarrhea, inflammation, chronic fatigue, diagnosed autoimmune disease, food allergies, or food intolerances. It has also been linked to medications such as aspirin and nonsteroidal anti-inflammatory drugs, which can irritate the bowel lining.

Lifestyle modification, including changing the diet and reducing stress, may be the best ways to treat leaky gut syndrome. Glutamine, an amino acid that can be taken in supplement form, may also protect the lining of the intestines, but clinical research is lacking and more results are needed in order to understand glutamine's effect on digestion. Probiotics also can be added to your diet in order to balance healthy gut bacteria. Foods such as yogurt, kefir, or fermented foods can all help restore balance among healthy gut bacteria.

Malabsorption Syndrome

Malabsorption syndrome is the direct result of another disease or disorder that causes the intestines to not properly absorb certain nutrients. These diseases include gastrointestinal diseases, such as Crohn's and celiac disease, but also AIDS/HIV, chronic liver disease, and treatment from radiation, certain types of cancer, parasitic infections, and some medications.

When any of these diseases or disorders occurs, the small intestine is damaged and inflamed. Since proteins, carbohydrates, fats, and fluids are absorbed in the small intestine, a person with any of these disorders will most likely suffer from malabsorption syndrome because the intestines simply can't absorb those important nutrients and fluids. Many of these conditions also cause the body to be incapable of producing certain enzymes needed to digest food.

 NOTABLE INSIGHT

Traveling abroad to Southeast Asia, the Caribbean, and India can lead to malabsorption as in the case of tropical sprue. It is caused by toxins in foods, infection, or parasites and can lead to anemia, diarrhea, sore tongue, and weight loss.

Recognizing the signs and symptoms of malabsorption is crucial for people with these disorders. Some symptoms include low blood pressure, weight loss, fatty stools, fluid retention, bloating, diarrhea, anemia, and weight loss. Other risk factors can include excessive alcohol consumption, family history of cystic fibrosis, intestinal surgery, and travel to Southeast Asia, the Caribbean, and India. A diagnosis of malabsorption syndrome can be easily confirmed by a biopsy of the small intestine or through blood work.

The first steps to manage and treat malabsorption syndrome start with nutrient and fluid replacement. In extreme cases, hospitalization is sometimes necessary if sufficient nutrient loss occurs. Diet is key to recovery, and small meals should be eaten throughout the day. The recovery diet should be rich in carbohydrates, fats, minerals, proteins, and vitamins. It's also important to stay hydrated.

NOTABLE INSIGHT

One easy way to recognize if you're drinking enough fluids is to look at the color of your urine. It should be the color of light yellow lemonade.

Gut Support with Probiotics

A healthy GI tract contains trillions of healthy or "good" bacteria, which help maintain a natural balance between healthy and unhealthy bacteria. Probiotics are healthy bacteria, and live cultures are found in fermented dairy products and foods. Yogurt and kefir typically contain *lactobacillus, bifidobacteria,* and other strains. These healthy bacteria may help strengthen your immune system, reduce the risk of certain cancers, decrease inflammation as with IBS, and help with other non-specific forms of diarrhea.

Prebiotics are nondigestible carbohydrates, such as plant fiber, that assist in growth of existing bacteria in the colon. Oligosaccharides and inulin are common types. When the naturally occurring healthy bacteria are out of balance due to long-term use of antibiotics or poor diet, it's a good idea to replenish the good bacteria. Fermented foods that contain probiotics, such as yogurt and kimchi, along with prebiotics like legumes, whole grains, and garlic, are good choices.

Water: An Essential Nutrient

Water is part of every chemical reaction that takes place in the body. You can only survive for about a week without water as opposed to several weeks without food. The function of water is to transport nutrients, oxygen, and waste throughout the body. It also helps to regulate body temperature, lubricate joints, protect organs, and relieve constipation.

The majority of water in the body can be divided into cellular and intracellular. Cellular water is found inside the cells, and intracellular water is found between the cells. Water helps facilitate the movement of molecules. The human body weight ranges from 45 to 75 percent water depending on age, sex, and level of body fat. Infants are about 75 percent water. An obese person with higher body fat will have less water than those with high muscle content.

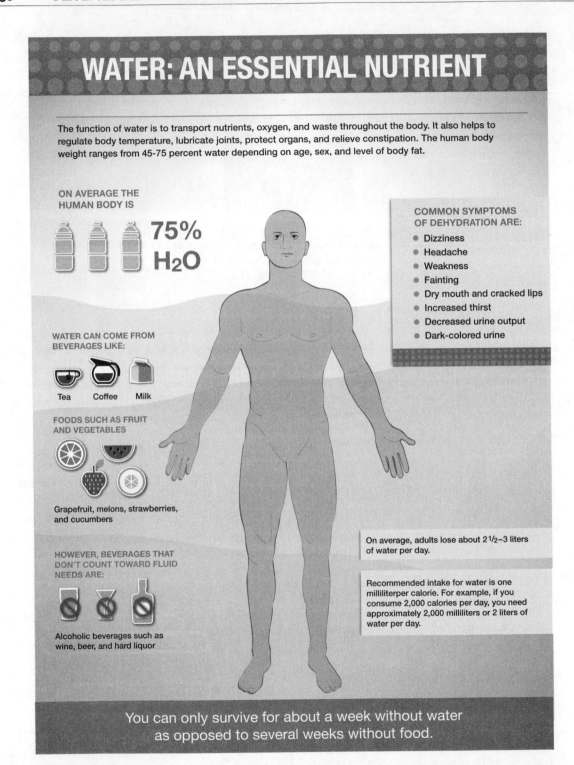

WATER: AN ESSENTIAL NUTRIENT

The function of water is to transport nutrients, oxygen, and waste throughout the body. It also helps to regulate body temperature, lubricate joints, protect organs, and relieve constipation. The human body weight ranges from 45-75 percent water depending on age, sex, and level of body fat.

ON AVERAGE THE HUMAN BODY IS

75% H_2O

WATER CAN COME FROM BEVERAGES LIKE:

Tea   Coffee   Milk

FOODS SUCH AS FRUIT AND VEGETABLES

Grapefruit, melons, strawberries, and cucumbers

HOWEVER, BEVERAGES THAT DON'T COUNT TOWARD FLUID NEEDS ARE:

Alcoholic beverages such as wine, beer, and hard liquor

COMMON SYMPTOMS OF DEHYDRATION ARE:
- Dizziness
- Headache
- Weakness
- Fainting
- Dry mouth and cracked lips
- Increased thirst
- Decreased urine output
- Dark-colored urine

On average, adults lose about 2 1/2–3 liters of water per day.

Recommended intake for water is one milliliterper calorie. For example, if you consume 2,000 calories per day, you need approximately 2,000 milliliters or 2 liters of water per day.

You can only survive for about a week without water as opposed to several weeks without food.

On average, adults lose about 2¹/₂ to 3 liters of water per day. Water loss can occur through regular bodily functions such as maintaining body temperature, sweating, going to the bathroom, and breathing.

Fluid homeostasis in your body is regulated very closely. It involves the kidneys, lungs, liver, adrenal glands, and the thirst centers of your brain. Each works in conjunction with the other to release hormones and electrolytes in order to maintain the fluid stores.

Recommended intake for water is 1 milliliter per calorie. For example, if you consume 2,000 calories per day, you need approximately 2,000 milliliters or 2 liters of water per day. Of course, this amount varies based on your activity level and your environment.

Common symptoms of dehydration are dizziness, headache, weakness, fainting, dry mouth and cracked lips, increased thirst, decreased urine output, and dark-colored urine.

Water is an essential nutrient for your body and it's important to consume an adequate amount each day. Most fluids you drink will count toward your fluid goals. Water from beverages like coffee, tea, and milk can count toward your goal, too. Highly caffeinated beverages can cause a slight increase in fluid output, but the body quickly adjusts.

The only beverages that don't count toward fluid needs are alcoholic beverages such as wine, beer, and hard liquor. These have a diuretic effect and promote the production of urine. It's a good idea to drink one glass of water per alcoholic beverage to maintain your hydration levels. Foods such as fruit and vegetables contain water, too. Some are even considered to have high water content, such as cucumbers, melons, strawberries, and grapefruit. Other foods like soup can also count toward your daily needs.

 WAKE-UP CALL

When increasing high-fiber foods in your diet, it's important to drink more water. Some fibrous foods absorb water and can cause an unpleasant experience in the bathroom: constipation.

Can You Drink Too Much Water?

Overconsumption of water is rare. A person would have to drink 10 to 20 liters of water over several hours, which would lower the sodium levels in the body and cause hyponatremia. This condition would lead to swelling of the brain, coma, convulsions, and possibly even death. Individuals at the greatest risk are endurance athletes, those with mental illnesses such as schizophrenia, and infants who receive only water instead of formula.

The Least You Need to Know

- Digestion is a complex process that allows you to absorb the vital nutrients from foods you eat.
- Food should never cause you pain. If pain is persistent, it can lead to serious digestive disorders and diseases. Be sure to seek medical help if this occurs.
- Include fermented foods such as yogurt, kimchi, and kefir in your diet to build up a healthy bacterial colony in your gut.
- Water is vital for good overall health. It's important to be sure to meet your water goal each day.

The Calorie

Where did the calorie originate? The calorie, as we recognize it today, originates from the eighteenth century. Wilbur Atwater, a pioneer in the field of nutrition, is the scientist credited with developing the "Atwater system," which was a means to measure the energy in food. His research was key in educating people about the importance of calories and their role in a healthy diet.

Everyone needs a certain amount of calories every day. Your body uses 60 percent of your total calories daily just to regulate itself while at rest. Another 10 percent are used in the digestion of food and absorption of nutrients. The remaining 30 percent are allotted for your activity needs. The U.S. Dietary Guidelines provide recommendations on how many calories you need each day based on your activity level, age, height, and gender. However, how your body metabolizes and burns those calories makes a huge impact on how easy or difficult it is to maintain your weight over your lifetime.

In This Chapter

- What is a calorie?
- How many calories do you need daily?
- Adjusting your calories to lose or gain weight
- Defining eating disorders
- Recognizing empty calories in your diet

The Origin of the Calorie

A calorie is a unit of measure. It is actually the amount of heat required to raise 1 kilogram of water 1° Celsius.

Let's say you want to know how many calories are in an apple. A scientist would place the apple in a metal chamber, which is contained within another insulated metal chamber of water. This device, known as a bomb calorimeter, measures the amount of heat released from the apple when it's cooked down to ashes. The measurements of the heat exchanged within the water are recorded and the data reveals that an apple provides about 93 calories.

Fortunately, the U.S. Department of Agriculture (USDA) maintains the food database that houses all the information about the nutrients specific foods contain, such as calories, vitamins, and minerals. The USDA has been collecting and analyzing data for more than 100 years, and with each new year more information is added.

What we have come to know as a "calorie" is technically a kilocalorie, which is equivalent to 1,000 calories. A kilocalorie contains enough energy to increase the temperature of 1 kilogram of water by 1° Celsius at sea level. A kilogram contains 1,000 grams and a kilocalorie contains 1,000 real calories. We simply refer to it as a calorie instead of the more accurate term kilocalorie or kcal.

Calories are found in carbohydrates, proteins, and fats. These are referred to as energy calories. Carbohydrates and proteins provide 4 calories per gram, fats provide 9 calories per gram, and alcohol provides 7 calories per gram.

 FOODIE FACTOID

Take a look at the calorie differences between the foods listed below. Fat and sugar provide the most calories in a small amount without any other nutrients besides energy calories. For example, a chicken breast and green beans provide much fewer calories by weight with an added bonus of valuable nutrients your body can use, such as proteins, vitamins, and minerals. It's important to be aware where the majority of your calories come from.

- 1 ounce of butter = 203 calories
- 1 ounce of sugar = 110 calories
- 1 ounce of chicken breast = 47 calories
- 1 ounce of green beans = 10 calories

Most foods contain a combination of carbohydrates, proteins, and fats, and it's easy to calculate the total calories of a food item. If you know that a cup of dry cereal contains 15 grams of carbohydrate, 3 grams of protein, and 1 gram of fat, you would simply multiply it by the appropriate amount of calories per gram for each nutrient.

For example:

> 15 grams of carbohydrates × 4 calories per gram = 60 calories
>
> 3 grams of protein × 4 calories per gram = 12 calories
>
> 1 gram of fat × 9 calories per gram = 9 calories
>
> 60 + 12 + 9 = 81 total calories

The energy nutrients provide calories or fuel for your body to run on. However, in addition to energy, we use carbohydrates, protein, and fats as building blocks in the body, which we'll discuss in greater detail in later chapters. If you consume more calories than your body needs each day, the extra calories are conveniently stored for later use. Unfortunately, over time these stored calories become unwanted pounds.

The U.S. government has established an estimated energy requirement (EER) to ensure we consume an adequate amount of energy each day to maintain health and ward off disease. Below is the table of estimated calorie requirements from the USDA Dietary Guidelines for Americans reported in 2010.

Estimated Calorie Needs per Day by Age, Gender, and Physical Activity Level

Gender	Age (years)	Sedentary	Moderately Active	Active
Child (female/male)	2-3	1,000-1,200	1,000-1,400	1,000-1,400
Female	4-8	1,200-1,400	1,400-1,600	1,400-1,800
	9-13	1,400-1,600	1,600-2,000	1,800-2,200
	14-18	1,800	2,000	2,400
	19-30	1,800-2,000	2,000-2,200	2,400
	31-50	1,800	2,000	2,400
	51+	1,600	1,800	2,000-2,200
Male	4-8	1,200-1,400	1,400-1,600	1,600-2,000
	9-13	1,600-2,000	1,800-2,200	2,000-2,600
	14-18	2,000-2,400	2,400-2,800	2,800-3,200
	19-30	2,400-2,600	2,600-2,800	3,000
	31-50	2,200-2,400	2,400-2,600	2,800-3,000
	51+	2,000-2,200	2,200-2,400	2,400-2,800

By glancing at the table you can see that as we age, we need fewer calories. Combine this with decreased activity levels and it's very easy to quickly add unwanted pounds after middle age.

How to Calculate Your Calories

To calculate your basal metabolic rate (BMR), you need to know your current weight in pounds, height in inches, and age. Next take your numbers and plug them into the Harris Benedict equation, which will give you the total calories your body needs at rest.

How to Calculate Your Basal Metabolic Rate

Women: 655 + (4.35 × weight in pounds) + (4.7 × height in inches) − (4.7 × age in years)

Men: 665 + (6.23 × weight in pounds) + (12.7 × height in inches)- (6.8 × age in years)

Example: a 40-year-old woman, who is 5'6" tall and weighs 176 pounds

655 + (4.35 × 176) + (4.7 × 66) - (4.7 × 40)

655 + 756.5 + 310.2 − 188 = 1,533.7 calories

Now let's calculate your activity factor by utilizing the following chart. Multiply your BMR by your activity factor to determine your total calorie needs for the day to maintain your current weight.

Activity Factors

Activity Level	Activity Factor
No exercise—mostly sitting	1.2
Light exercise (1-3 days per week)	1.375
Moderate exercise (3-5 days per week)	1.55
Heavy exercise (6-7 days per week)	1.725

Example: BMR 1,533.7 × 1.2 (no exercise) = 1,840.44 calories

Knowing your body's total calorie needs will help you achieve your weight goals.

Basal Metabolism Rate (BMR)

Your basal metabolism rate accounts for about 60 percent of your daily energy needs. The body uses these calories while it's at rest to carry out all types of key functions you don't have to think about, such as breathing, pumping blood, and making new cells. BMRs vary between men and women because men have more lean muscle mass and muscle is metabolically active (burns more energy).

As you age, your BMR will decrease by about 2 percent per decade. This is due to a change in hormone levels, body composition changes such as a decrease in lean muscle mass, and decreased activity level.

Your BMR can also be negatively affected if you've followed very low-calorie diets and skipped meals for many years, which causes your body to hold tightly to its calorie stores by utilizing calories more efficiently. We'll discuss this in more detail shortly.

Cutting Calories for Weight Loss

One pound of body fat is equivalent to 3,500 calories. According to a review of research published in *Strategies to Prevent Weight Gain Among Adults,* most people will gain 1 to 2 pounds each year in middle age. This is a slow and gradual increase over a long period of time, which can lead to obesity along with an increased risk of heart disease, hypertension, and diabetes.

An awareness of what your daily calorie needs are and a sensible approach to reducing calories for weight loss is the key to good health. The first step in cutting calories for weight loss is to create a calorie deficit each week through diet and exercise. First, determine whether you want to promote a half-pound or a whole pound of weight loss each week. A half-pound calorie deficit would equal 250 calories per day. A one-pound loss would require a 500 calorie deficit. Next, you would deduct 250 to 500 calories from your total daily calories to determine your calorie budget for the day to promote weight loss.

For example, if your total daily calories were 1,840, to maintain your weight you would subtract 500 calories from your total: 1,840 - 500 = 1,340 calories. Next, you want to distribute those 1,500 calories throughout the day into three meals: breakfast, lunch, and dinner, and two snacks. A good plan would be to have 350 calories at breakfast, 350 calories at lunch, and 350 calories at dinner, with two snacks of 145 calories each in between meals.

You may realize that by implementing this regimen with more frequent meals, it seems to be much more food than you typically have been eating—and it may very well be. By eating frequent meals, you'll help stave off hunger and regularly fuel your body. Keep in mind that your body uses about 10 percent of its total calories to digest and assimilate food, so you might just be getting a slight metabolic increase from what you were previously.

NOTABLE INSIGHT

Researchers at Cornell University observed students' food selections after an 18-hour fast and found that vegetables were last on the list. Most were drawn to the higher-calorie foods such as starches and proteins, and they proceeded to eat more or overeat in that category.

Earlier we stated that muscle is metabolically active, meaning it burns more calories at rest. If you exercise and build more lean muscle mass in your body, you're going to increase the total amount of weight lost each week. By pairing eating fewer calories along with increased calorie burn from activity, you have a winning combination. There are no tools or exercise equipment required to be more active. All you need is a good pair of comfortable walking shoes—in a brisk 30-minute walk, you can burn off about 100 additional calories.

What Is an Empty Calorie?

Some calories are referred to as "empty" calories. This is a misnomer because there aren't really any calorie-free whole foods. An empty calorie is one in which the majority of calories are from sugary or fatty foods that don't provide any additional vitamins or minerals. This includes alcoholic beverages, too. Examples of empty-calorie foods include ice cream, candies, cookies, sodas and energy drinks, alcohol, and hot dogs.

Many people fill up on these types of foods and have no room left to eat more nutritious ones. The good news is when you eliminate these empty-calorie food sources from your diet you have more calories to use on healthier food options. Having some empty calories in your diet is allowable, but it should fit within your calorie budget.

One area where calories can add up quickly is with alcoholic beverages. Over the course of an evening, you could easily rack up an extra 300 calories with just a couple of drinks.

- 12 ounces of beer = 148 calories

- 1½ ounces of vodka (80 proof) = 96 calories

- 5 ounces of cabernet = 124 calories

- 3⅓ ounces of margarita = 153 calories

- 10 ounces of Bloody Mary = 125 calories

Your best low-calorie choices are light beer at 95 calories, $1^1/_2$ ounces of hard liquor with a zero-calorie mixer, or a glass of wine. Be wary of mixed drinks and know your calorie budget when including cocktails.

How Healthy Is Your Body Weight?

Determining whether you're at a healthy weight is important for good health. However, keep in mind that numbers are just that, and they don't show the whole health picture. It's important to take everything into consideration when assessing your health status: genetics, BMI, frame size, muscle and fat percentages, and location of your body fat, along with an evaluation of your blood lipid levels.

Research from the Centers for Disease Control and Prevention (CDC) shows that those who live the longest are actually considered to be in the "overweight" and "mildly obese" categories. The studies suggest that people with a BMI of 25 to 29.9 may outlive those with higher and lower BMIs.

Body Mass Index (BMI)

Body mass index (BMI) is a calculation used by many health practitioners to determine if a person is at a healthy weight based on their weight-to-height ratio. It helps them gauge the risk of disease as related to weight status. Some of the criticism over the use of this measure is that it was based on healthy population studies and doesn't take into consideration that women have more body fat than men, older people have more body fat than younger adults, and athletes have a higher muscle mass.

To calculate your BMI, you take your weight in pounds divided by height in inches squared × 703. For example, let's say you are 150 pounds and 5'7":

150 pounds ÷ 67 × 67 inches × 703 = 23.49

BMI = 23

 WAKE-UP CALL

You can determine your risk of heart attack if you're over 20 years old and don't have heart disease or diabetes by using the heart attack risk assessment and BMI calculator provided at the following websites:

Heart Attack Risk Calculator:

- heart.org/HEARTORG/Conditions/HeartAttack/HeartAttackToolsResources/Heart-Attack-Risk-Assessment_UCM_303944_Article.jsp

BMI Calculator

- nhlbi.nih.gov/health/educational/lose_wt/BMI/bmicalc.htm

BMI Ranges

BMI	Weight Status
Below 18.5	Underweight
18.5–25.0	Normal weight
25.0–30.0	Overweight
30.0 and above	Obese

BMI is an inexpensive and quick gauge of health as opposed to other more complicated methods to evaluate the fat level. Additional methods to determine levels of body fat are more expensive, require trained staff, and are not all portable. These include skin-fold measures taken with calipers, underwater weighing, bioelectrical impedance, and dual-energy x-ray absorptiometry (DXA).

BMIs can be higher than 35. A BMI of 40 or more is considered severe obesity or morbidly obese, which equates to about 100 pounds over your ideal body weight. However, you can be classified as morbidly obese if you have a BMI of 35 and the presence of obesity-related health issues such as diabetes or high blood pressure.

Long-Term Weight Management

According to a report by the National Health and Nutrition Examination Survey (NHANES), over 70 percent of Americans have a BMI greater than 25, which classifies them as overweight or obese. Individuals categorized as overweight or obese have an increased risk of developing conditions and diseases such as high cholesterol, diabetes, hypertension, metabolic disorders, and heart disease.

Distribution of fat is a critical component in assessing the risk factor for developing certain metabolic disorders. Carrying weight in the lower portion of the body, primarily the hip and buttocks region, is called *gynoid* or "pear" shape. If an individual carries their body weight around their middle or abdominal area, they have an *android* or "apple" shape. The apple style of weight distribution generally denotes an increased amount of internal fat, known as visceral fat, around the organs. Visceral fat increases the risk for hypertension, heart disease, and type 2 diabetes.

Treating weight gain involves a combination of exercise, diet, and behavior modification. Environment is an important component of behavior modification. Factors in the environment can trigger the desire to eat, such as the smell and sight of food. These factors can also trigger the selection of types and quantities of food. Social cues such as food selection of dining partners and cognitive cues like how you feel about food can also affect your behavior.

Setting a realistic weight-loss goal is crucial. Endotext, a nonprofit web-based source of information on endocrine disease, recommends a 10 percent weight-loss goal over 6 months as a realistic reduction. By focusing on a weekly goal of losing 1 to 2 pounds, you should achieve your 10 percent goal within a 6-month period. The National Weight Control Registry reports individuals who monitor their weight closely with frequent weigh-ins (daily to weekly) are able to modify their behavior instantly and achieve better results than those who did not weigh in on a frequent basis.

Reducing daily calorie intake by 250 to 500 calories and making small changes is key to changing your behavior. Endotext reports individuals who reduce their calorie intake and limit their fat intake to 20 to 30 percent of their ingested calories had greater success in weight reduction than calorie or fat reduction alone.

When you decrease your calorie intake, you will likely lose weight. Losing weight is followed by *adaptive thermogenesis*. Your body has less of you to move and therefore requires fewer calories. This is why increasing activity levels is important for ongoing weight loss and management.

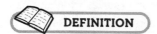

DEFINITION

Thermogenesis is energy produced from the breakdown and processing of the food you eat. **Adaptive thermogenesis** is when your body regulates the production of heat (burning of calories) in response to environmental changes in temperature and diet, which causes metabolic inefficiency.

Eating More for Weight Gain

Trying to gain weight can be just as big of a hurdle as losing weight. It requires the same amount of dedication to achieve your weight goals. In order to gain 1 to 2 pounds per week, take your total calorie needs for the day and increase them by 500 to 1,000 calories. Distribute the 500 to 1,000 calories over each meal and snack times. For example, if your calorie requirements are 2,000 per day, add 100 to 200 calories at each mealtime. You can easily add an extra 100 calories to your diet by eating $1/4$ cup of granola, 1 cup of air-popped popcorn, 1 ounce of cheddar cheese, or 15 almonds.

Eating Disorders

When eating (or the lack of eating) becomes such a personal obsession that it disrupts normal daily living, an eating disorder is most likely the cause. According to the National Association of Anorexia Nervosa and Associated Disorders, about 24 million people suffer from an eating disorder. The primary types of eating disorders are anorexia nervosa, bulimia, and binge eating. Each disorder revolves around extreme emotions, behaviors, and attitudes toward food. Becoming preoccupied with food and weight is a sign that an eating disorder may be present.

Multiple psychological and neurochemical factors lead to eating disorders. Disordered eating is prevalent among athletes due to weight requirements for certain sports like gymnastics and wrestling. These disorders can lead to serious life-threatening health issues, and more people die from eating disorders when compared to other forms of mental illness.

Anorexia Nervosa

Anorexia, as it is commonly referred to, is when a person eats too little food to maintain a healthy weight. A person with anorexia has an intense fear of weight gain and a distorted body image, which is linked to self-esteem. Anorexia affects about $1/2$ to 1 percent of girls or women, according to the National Eating Disorders Organization.

Some of the key warning signs of anorexia nervosa are extreme weight loss, preoccupation with weight and dieting practices, avoidance of certain foods, constant references to being overweight, excessive exercising, and withdrawal from social situations. Those who suffer from anorexia not only restrict food, but they can also binge and purge on foods to control body weight. Severe food restriction can cause muscle wasting, hair loss, and overall malnutrition.

Treatment for anorexia involves psychological and nutritional counseling. In extreme cases, an in-patient approach is necessary with 24-hour supervision in a specialized treatment facility. Of those who are diagnosed, between 5 and 20 percent die from the disorder.

Bulimia

Bulimia is an eating disorder characterized by repeatedly eating large amounts of food and then purging the food with self-induced vomiting or use of laxatives, along with excessive exercise to prevent weight gain. It affects 1 to 2 percent of adolescent and young adult women. A person with this type of eating disorder feels out of control and has self-esteem issues related to body image.

Some of the warning signs of bulimia are swelling of the cheeks or jaws, discoloration of teeth, rigid exercise routines, and frequent trips to the bathroom after meals. This disease adversely impacts the body by the repeated use of vomiting, which damages the gastrointestinal tract and disrupts the body's natural fluid balance. Treatment involves psychological and nutritional counseling along with antidepressants.

Binge-Eating Disorder (BED)

Binge-eating disorder (BED) is characterized by consuming large amounts of food in a very short period of time. A person with this type of eating disorder will typically binge in private and experience extreme feelings of guilt, shame, and being out of control during the episode. According to the National Eating Disorder Organization, it affects 1 to 5 percent of people in the

United States, with about 60 percent being female and only 40 percent male. Those with BED can be of average weight or classified as overweight.

Symptoms include frequent consumption of large amounts of foods in private, depression, eating until it hurts, and managing weight gain through self-induced vomiting. Repeated binge-eating episodes can lead to obesity along with obesity-related diseases, such as heart disease, diabetes, gallbladder disease, and high blood pressure. Treatment typically involves psychotherapy, nutritional counseling, and antidepressants.

Orthorexia

A relatively new eating disorder, orthorexia is not classified in the *Diagnostic and Statistical Manual of Mental Disorders (DSM)*. Introduced by Dr. Steven Bratman in 1997, orthorexia is closely related to anorexia nervosa. However, anorexics want to control weight, whereas in people with orthorexia, weight is not the focus. In orthorexia, a person has an obsession with eating "healthy" foods. The focus is on food quality, purity, and wholesomeness, along with avoidance of chemicals like preservatives or animal products. The consequences of this can lead to malnutrition and being underweight.

People affected by orthorexia may have started out by changing their eating habits to become healthier. However, the diet spirals out of control and turns into an obsession. These people may spend hours reading food labels, are preoccupied with how eating an "impure" food will impact their health, and also may believe they're better than other people for following such a "perfect" diet. Recovery is possible for those suffering from orthorexia. Treatment is similar to anorexia and involves psychological and nutritional counseling.

Tracking Your Calories

There are many ways to track your calories and monitor your progress when it comes to losing or gaining weight. Many people use the pen and paper method of a food log in which they write down what they ate, when they ate, and the estimated calories of each meal. Others may prefer to use a digital version. In today's electronic realm, there are even apps to help you keep track of your calories. Some apps even let you take photos of what you eat with your phone or tablet and the software calculates, tracks, and graphs your progress in full color.

It's important to know where the majority of your calories are coming from because it makes you aware of areas for improvement. You may learn that your meals are out of balance and don't have a healthy ratio of carbohydrates, proteins, and fats. It also helps identify if you are eating too much or too little which can cause unwanted weight gain or weight loss. It's hard to make changes in your diet if you don't know what you've been doing. And with today's technology at your fingertips it makes calculating calories easy. Knowing your total calorie needs for the day, how many calories you need to maintain your weight, and your BMI can help define your health goals and lead to better health.

You also need to be mindful and realize that counting calories should be used as a tool to help guide your towards making healthier, well-balanced food choices. When the numbers get in the way of the joy of eating there may be an underlying disordered way of eating present that needs to be addressed.

The Least You Need to Know

- A calorie is a measure of energy in food.
- The location of your body fat can adversely affect your health.
- Calories are not considered "good" or "bad."
- When eating or dieting becomes an obsession, it can lead to serious health risks.
- Men burn more calories at rest than women, due to a higher percentage of muscle mass.
- To maintain a healthy weight, it's important to be aware of how many calories you're ingesting.

Carbohydrates

Carbohydrates provide energy for your body, which is why the bulk of the calories in your diet should come from carbs. Every cell in your body can use the simple sugar molecule—glucose derived from carbohydrates. Without an adequate intake of carbohydrates, your nervous system, kidneys, muscles, and brain can't function properly. It is unfortunate that many people don't understand the critical role of carbohydrates in the body and just how important they are for a healthy body.

In this chapter, we look at the impact carbohydrates have on our diet, sort out the facts about simple and complex carbohydrates, and discuss the different types of fiber and where to find them.

In This Chapter

- What is a carbohydrate?
- The important role of carbohydrates in the body
- Distinguishing between simple and complex carbohydrates
- Identifying the best types of carbohydrates for good health
- The many benefits of soluble and insoluble fiber
- A quick review of sugar substitutes

Fuel for Your Body

A carbohydrate is referred to as an energy nutrient because it provides 4 calories per gram. Structurally, it's made up of carbon, oxygen, and hydrogen molecules. Recommendations for carbohydrate requirements are based on the minimum amount required for your body to properly function. The brain needs 50 to 100 grams of carbohydrate per day. Generally your diet should contain about 45 to 65 percent carbohydrates.

Carbohydrates are classified as simple or complex. There are also sugar alcohols and sugar substitutes, which are derivatives of carbohydrates. Foods high in carbohydrates tend to get oversimplified and labeled as "good" or "bad." This unfortunate labeling leads people to avoid them when they change their eating habits. Most people think of bread, pasta, and sugar when they think of the word "carbohydrates." Additionally, many people don't realize that fiber is a complex carbohydrate, too.

Carbohydrates get broken down in the body to their simplest forms, a one-sugar molecule called glucose. Glucose is the preferred source of energy for your body, brain, and red blood cells. Your body can also store glucose, but first must transform it to what is called glycogen. About a third of glycogen resides in the liver. The liver also coverts the glycogen to glucose and releases it into the blood. Muscle tissue contains glycogen stores, too, which is what gives an athlete an extra burst of energy. In fact, carbohydrates are so important to your body that when there's an insufficient amount of carbohydrates coming from your diet to sustain your body's needs, it's capable of using an alternate plan for generating energy from fat called *ketogenesis*. There are also times when your body encounters problems utilizing energy from glucose, as happens with diabetes.

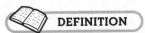 **DEFINITION**

> **Ketogenesis** is the breakdown of fat due to an inadequate supply of carbohydrates. Fragments of broken fats combine to form ketone bodies, which are used instead of glucose. They can alter the body's pH and cause dehydration, headaches, weakness, and irritability.

How Carbohydrates Are Broken Down by the Body

Carbohydrate digestion begins as soon as you place a carbohydrate-containing food into your mouth. Your salivary glands release a digestive enzyme called amylase, which helps break down a carbohydrate into smaller units of sugars. You can actually taste the action of amylase in your mouth. Simply take a small piece of white bread and hold it on your tongue. As saliva moistens the bread, you can taste it getting sweeter as it dissolves.

A carbohydrate is a combination of molecules called saccharides. A saccharide is sugar. Because food spends a short time in your mouth, only a few one-sugar molecules are released from the foods called *monosaccharides*. After foods are swallowed, the enzymes continue working to break apart the sugars even as they pass through your esophagus into the stomach. Amylase action ends only when the stomach acid becomes too concentrated.

In the stomach, the monosaccharides are further broken down by hydrochloric acid (HCL), which is naturally present in your stomach. Starches are also broken down, but there are no enzymes present in your stomach to break down those sugars or any fiber that may be present.

 NOTABLE INSIGHT

> Carbohydrates are easily digested and absorbed. Your body can digest a carbohydrate in 15 minutes to 1 hour.

As the food is released from your stomach into your small intestine in small, teaspoon-size amounts, the pancreas releases pancreatic amylase through a duct. Amylase aids in digestion of the polysaccharides and breaks them down into shorter and shorter chains of glucose and maltose. Maltase functions to break down starches into altose.

Monosaccharides like glucose are transported to the liver through your bloodstream. The liver regulates blood glucose levels and maintains it between 80 to 120 mg/DL. The liver can also store blood glucose in the form of glycogen for later use. Only enough can be stored to last for 10 to 18 hours. Galactose and fructose will also be metabolized by the liver and used by the liver for energy or to make other substances.

What is not absorbed is fiber, which moves on into the large intestine. The large intestine contains bacteria, which use the food leftovers to help produce some vitamins and also help break down and ferment fiber.

The Many Faces of Carbohydrates

There are many different types of saccharides, depending on how many saccharide units are linked together. These include mono-, di-, oligo-, and polysaccharides. The name is a clue as to how many saccharide units there are—mono- equals 1 unit, di- equals 2, oligo- equals 3 to 10, and poly- means many. The mono- and disaccharides are classified as simple carbohydrates. The oligo- and polysaccharides are classified as complex carbohydrates.

FOOD, GLUCOSE, AND THE BODY

Carbohydrate digestion begins as soon as you place a carbohydrate-containing food into your mouth.

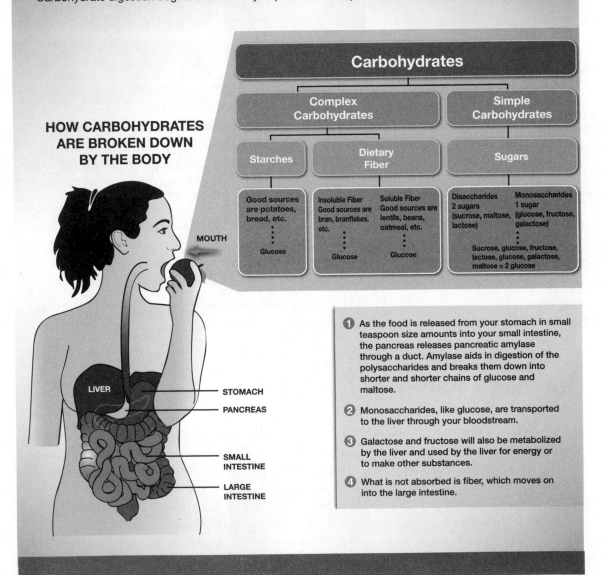

HOW CARBOHYDRATES ARE BROKEN DOWN BY THE BODY

Carbohydrates

Complex Carbohydrates		Simple Carbohydrates
Starches	Dietary Fiber	Sugars

Good sources are potatoes, bread, etc.
⋮
Glucose

Insoluble Fiber Good sources are bran, branflakes, etc.
⋮
Glucose

Soluble Fiber Good sources are lentils, beans, oatmeal, etc.
⋮
Glucose

Disaccharides 2 sugars (sucrose, maltose, lactose)

Monosaccharides 1 sugar (glucose, fructose, galactose)

⋮
Sucrose, glucose, fructose, lactose, glucose, galactose, maltose = 2 glucose

MOUTH

LIVER
STOMACH
PANCREAS
SMALL INTESTINE
LARGE INTESTINE

1 As the food is released from your stomach in small teaspoon size amounts into your small intestine, the pancreas releases pancreatic amylase through a duct. Amylase aids in digestion of the polysaccharides and breaks them down into shorter and shorter chains of glucose and maltose.

2 Monosaccharides, like glucose, are transported to the liver through your bloodstream.

3 Galactose and fructose will also be metabolized by the liver and used by the liver for energy or to make other substances.

4 What is not absorbed is fiber, which moves on into the large intestine.

Simple Carbohydrates

The simplest forms of sugar are monosaccharides and disaccharides. The monosaccharides are glucose, fructose, and galactose, and they're classified as simple carbohydrates. Glucose is the preferred sugar of your brain and body. Fructose is found in fruit and honey. It's slightly sweeter than table sugar, which is sucrose. Galactose is a milk sugar.

Disaccharides are two simple sugars bonded together. These are sucrose, lactose, and maltose. Sucrose is made of glucose and fructose, and it's the most common in our diets. Lactose is comprised of glucose and galactose, which is found in dairy products. Maltose consists of two glucose molecules.

The Glycemic Response to Carbohydrates

The glycemic index refers to a food's ability to increase your blood glucose levels. Refined carbohydrates like white bread and fruit juice can be easily absorbed by your body. Research suggests there's a possible relationship between consuming high-glycemic foods and obesity, as well as an increased risk of type 2 diabetes and coronary heart disease. The criticism of the glycemic load is that we don't generally eat single food items like white bread at meals. We eat a mixed meal composed of many foods, which will alter the glycemic load.

The glycemic index is determined by the increase in blood glucose during a two hour period after consumption of a certain amount of carbohydrates as compared to an equal amount of carbohydrates from a reference food. The higher the glycemic load, the higher the expected rise in glucose. Complex carbohydrates that are high in fiber will always have a lower glycemic index.

Sugar Alcohols

Sugar alcohols are derived from sugar found in fruits and berries. However, these sugars are chemically altered in the lab and therefore only provide 2 calories per gram. They don't have a direct impact on blood sugar. However, because they're a type of carbohydrate, if too much is consumed, they will eventually raise blood sugar levels.

The food industry can use sugar alcohols as thickeners or as sweeteners. Typically, they're combined with other sugar substitutes. You can find sugar alcohols in diabetic foods, chewing gums, and hard candies. A high consumption of foods containing sugar alcohols will lead to bloating and diarrhea due to the fact that they are not completely absorbed in the digestive tract, and they will ferment, causing a laxative effect along with gas and bloating. Xylitol, mannitol, and sorbitol are all examples of sugar alcohols. Xylitol is as sweet as sugar and can be used in a 1:1 replacement. Be sure to closely read food labels, as items labeled "diabetic," "sugar free," or "no sugar added" may contain sugar alcohols.

Sugar Substitutes

Sugar substitutes entered the marketplace in the 1950s. Popularity has risen in response to people's desire to decrease calories without sacrificing flavor. Because they don't adversely impact blood sugar, sugar substitutes are popular with people with diabetes. They may be referred to as nonnutritive sweeteners, artificial sweeteners, and very low-calorie sweeteners.

The FDA regulates artificial sweeteners and has established an acceptable daily intake (ADI) for sucralose, saccharin, and acesulfame K to prevent health risks. However, you would have to consume the sweeteners in copious amounts to exceed recommendations. If you are following a healthy diet, you would automatically be consuming very little added sugars, whether they be all natural or made in a lab.

The food industry tends to blend a variety of these sweeteners to improve the overall taste profile in food products and help negate any aftertaste. Be sure to check your food labels to identify which ones you're consuming. Check out the following list for a few of the common sugar substitutes available in the marketplace.

- **Sucralose (Splenda):** Made from chemically altered sugar, it passes through the GI tract undigested and unabsorbed. It's 600 times sweeter than sugar. The product has various blends that can be used as a 1:1 replacement in baked goods and as a tabletop sweetener. It's also used in carbonated beverages and desserts.

- **Stevia (Truvia and SweetLeaf):** Made from the leaves of an herb that looks similar to the mint plant. It's 30 times sweeter than sugar and provides no calories or carbohydrates. It passes through the GI tract undigested and unabsorbed. It cannot be used in baked goods because it's not heat stable. However, they do offer variations that can be used in baking, such as Stevia Plus.

- **Agave Nectar:** Made from the same plant that's used for making tequila. It's a refined product and has a higher concentration of fructose than table sugar. It's 1.5 times sweeter than sugar and provides 60 calories per tablespoon as compared to sugar's 40 calories per tablespoon. Because it's sweeter, people find they need less of it to sweeten items, which makes it popular with diabetics. However, 1 tablespoon still has 15g of carbohydrates. It can be used as a sugar replacement in baking ($^2/_3$ cup agave to 1 cup sugar), but you must reduce the baking temperature by 25°F and reduce liquids by $^1/_4$ cup.

- **Saccharin (Sweet 'N Low):** Made from saccharin in the United States and sodium cyclamate in Canada. Saccharin passes through the GI tract undigested and unabsorbed. It's 10 times sweeter than sugar by weight and provides 4 calories per gram.

- **Acesulfame K (Sweet One/Sunnet):** Made from acesulfame potassium, it's 200 times sweeter than sugar and provides less than 4 calories per serving. It passes through the GI tract undigested and unabsorbed. It's heat stable and can be used in baking.

- **Aspartame (Nutrasweet/Equal)**: Made from aspartic acid, phenylalanine, and methanol. It's not safe for individuals with a rare genetic disorder phenylketonuria (PKU) as they are unable to break down the phenylalanine component. It is 200 times sweeter than sugar and provides 4 calories per serving. Its sweetness lasts longer than table sugar and it has a long shelf life. It is typically combined with acesulfame K. Aspartame can not be used in baking as it breaks down in high temperatures and in high pH.

It's a good idea to read food labels for added sugars. You may find these types of claims listed on products in the marketplace.

- **Sugar-free:** Less than 0.5 grams of sugar per serving.

- **Reduced sugar or less sugar:** At least 25 percent less sugar(s) per serving as compared to a standard serving of the traditional full-sugar food item.

- **No added sugars, without added sugar, no sugar:** No sugars are added during processing; contains no ingredients such as fruit juice.

FOODIE FACTOID

The suffix -ose at the end of a word denotes a sugar. The suffix -ase at the end of a word denotes an enzyme that breaks down a sugar.

Complex Carbohydrates

The complex carbohydrates are categorized as oligosaccharides or polysaccharides. Oligosaccharides contain short chains of monosaccharides linked together, such as raffinose, stachyose, verbascose, and maltodextrin.

Polysaccharides come from starch, glycogen, and fibers. Starch is the storage of glucose in plants. We use enzymes like amylase to help break down starch into smaller units of glucose. Starches are found in beans and legumes, whole grains, and vegetables. Fibers, which we will discuss next, are made up of monosaccharides. The primary source of fiber in our diets is plant cellulose.

Dietary Fiber

Dietary fiber is currently classified as soluble or insoluble. However, the Institute of Medicine (IOM) would like a third category added named functional fiber, which would include extracted fiber used as supplements. Humans are unable to digest fiber because they do not have the enzyme necessary to break it down for use in the body. Each type of fiber plays an important role in the body such as holding water, providing roughage, and reducing the risk of certain diseases. About 95 percent of fiber comes from the cell walls of plants. Most fiber is technically a nonstarch polysaccharide like cellulose, hemicelluloses, lignin, resistant starch, pectin, gums, and mucilages.

Soluble Fiber

Soluble fiber dissolves in water and forms a gel. When you cook a batch of oatmeal, you'll note how "gummy" it becomes. Soluble fiber also slows down digestion and makes you feel full. Bacteria in the colon can ferment soluble fiber. Soluble fiber also helps maintain blood sugar levels, which is important for people with diabetes. It also helps lower cholesterol levels when the gel-like substance passes through your intestine and traps cholesterol.

Gums are found in legumes, oatmeal, and beans. Pectin is found in fruit, apples, strawberries, oranges, and citrus. Fermentable fibers are primarily pectin and gums along with a few hemicelluloses. Hemicellulose is a group of complex carbohydrates that along with pectins surround the cellulose fibers of plant cells. These fibers help increase water and sodium absorption in the colon. They can also promote cell growth, increase acidity, and provide energy by breaking down short-chain fatty acids.

NOTABLE INSIGHT

When you go on a low-carbohydrate diet, it appears that you lose a few pounds within a day. However, much of that weight is water loss. As your glycogen stores are depleted, you lose water because each glycogen molecule contains about 2.7 grams of water.

Insoluble Fiber

Insoluble fiber doesn't dissolve in water and adds bulk to the foodstuff in your GI tract. This keeps things moving through your system by adding roughage, decreasing transit time, and making it easier for you to go to the bathroom. Bacteria in the colon don't easily ferment insoluble fibers. Foods that contain insoluble fiber such as cellulose are whole-wheat flour, bran, cabbage, peas, beans, and grains. Hemicellulose would be found in bran, cereal, and whole grains. Lignin is found in wheat and mature vegetables, such as in the skins of potatoes.

Functional Fiber

The term "functional fiber" refers to isolated, purified forms of nondigestible carbohydrates that have beneficial effects in humans. These are made from fiber extracted from plants or animals. Common types are psyllium, inulin, and oligofructose. These can be consumed in the form of pills or powders and added to food products.

How Much Fiber Do I Need?

It has been reported that Americans only consume about 15 grams of dietary fiber daily, which is not surprising since we don't get enough daily servings of fruits, vegetables, and whole grains in our diets. The IOM recommends 25 grams of fiber per day for women under 50 and teenage girls. Men under 50 should get 30 to 38 grams per day. Be sure to eat a combination of soluble and insoluble fiber.

 FOODIE FACTOID

Functional fiber may not be vegetarian. Lobster, crab, and shrimp shells are used to create chitosan, which is an indigestible modified carbohydrate polymer sold in supplements.

Discovering High-Fiber Foods

High-fiber foods are beneficial to your health. They're usually more nutrient-dense, will decrease your total calorie intake because you are eating fewer calories overall, and are typically lower in fat. Research has shown that diets high in fiber help maintain blood sugar levels in people with type 2 diabetes. Fiber aids in weight loss by making you feel fuller so you eat less. It can reduce heart disease risk by lowering total blood cholesterol levels. Fiber may also reduce the risk of cancer, hypertension, and gastrointestinal diseases.

Be sure to check the label when you look for fiber-rich foods at the store. The first word in an ingredient list of a fiber-rich grain should be "whole." To be considered a good source of fiber, a product should provide 5 or more grams per serving.

Get more fiber into your diet by adding whole-fiber foods at each meal. At breakfast, start with a whole-grain cereal and add berries. For lunch, use whole-grain breads to make sandwiches or add beans as a soup or a dip. At your evening meal, make vegetables the star. Snack time also makes a great place to add finger-friendly foods like carrots or the portable apple. Check out the fiber-rich foods in the following chart. It's easy to bulk up your diet with these fiber-rich foods.

Top 10 Fiber-Rich Foods

1 medium pear	5.1 grams
¹/₂ cup raspberries	4.0 grams
1 cup brussels sprouts	6.4 grams
1 cup broccoli	5.3 grams
¹/₂ cup peas	4.4 grams
¹/₂ cup black beans	7.5 grams
¹/₂ cup lentils	7.8 grams
1 cup barley	6.0 grams
1 cup quinoa	5.0 grams
1 cup oatmeal	4.0 grams

All vegetables and grains are cooked.

More Is Not Always Better

Now that you realize all the great benefits fiber has to offer, you'll want to add fiber-rich foods to your meals. It's a good idea to gradually increase your fiber over time. If you add too much too soon, your body will not be geared up to handle it. Remember, fiber is fermented in your colon and a byproduct of fermentation is gas production (methane). If you increase fibrous foods too fast, it will cause GI distress like excess gas and bloating. Add one high-fiber food at a time and see how your body handles it. If you can tolerate the new fiber-rich food, add another the next day and so on.

 FOODIE FACTOID

Epazote is a word derived from the Aztecs and means "skunk sweat." It's a green leafy herb with a flavor similar to anise and a smell like turpentine and citronella. It aids in the prevention of gas formation in the GI tract and is traditionally cooked with black beans.

High-Fiber Recipe

The following recipe is a great source of high fiber.

Raspberry Coconut Quinoa Breakfast Bowl

Move over oatmeal, quinoa is in the house! This sweet and savory breakfast bowl will energize you all the way to lunch.

Yield:	Prep Time:	Cook Time:	Serving Size:
4 servings	10 minutes	20 minutes	1 cup

Each serving has:			
280 calories	6g total fat	3g saturated fat	7g protein
52g carbohydrate	6g fiber	0mg cholesterol	95mg sodium

$1/2$ cup red quinoa

$1/2$ cup white quinoa

$1/4$ cup sweetened flaked coconut

$1/2$ cup light coconut milk, canned

1 TB. grated and peeled ginger

$1/4$ cup packed brown sugar

$1/8$ tsp. kosher salt

6 ounces raspberries

2 TB fresh mint, finely minced

1. Rinse quinoa in a fine strainer.

2. Combine 2 cups of water with 1 cup of mixed quinoa in a small saucepan.

3. Bring to a boil and reduce to a simmer. Cover saucepan with lid and cook quinoa for 15 minutes or until all water has been absorbed.

4. While quinoa is cooking, toast sweetened coconut in a small nonstick saucepan for 4 to 5 minutes over medium heat, stirring occasionally until golden brown in color. Set aside.

5. Combine coconut milk, ginger, brown sugar, and salt in a small bowl and pour over cooked quinoa.

6. Fold in raspberries.

7. Garnish with toasted coconut and mint.

Variation: Use any color of quinoa.

The Least You Need to Know

- Carbohydrates are used to make glucose, which is the preferred fuel for your body.

- Complex carbohydrates contain beneficial fiber.

- Eat the skins of fruits and vegetables to up your fiber intake.

- Fiber fills you up and can aid in weight loss.

- Limit your intake of added sugars for better health.

- Read food labels when you select foods that appear to be high in fiber to ensure they actually are a good source of fiber.

Protein

Protein is one of the three macronutrients along with fat and carbohydrates. The word *protein* comes from the Greek term for "primary," *proteios*. All macronutrients are "energy" nutrients that provide calories. Protein, just like carbohydrates, provides 4 calories per gram.

Each cell in your body contains protein and it is involved in the development, maintenance, and repair of the human body. In this chapter, we'll look at what protein is made of, how much you need each day, and examine its role in your body. We'll also discuss why consumption of complete proteins is important.

In This Chapter

- What is a protein?
- The function of amino acids in the body
- The process of protein digestion and absorption
- Complete and incomplete proteins
- How not eating enough protein affects health
- What happens if you eat more protein than your body needs?

The Building Blocks of the Body

Proteins are large molecules made up of strands of amino acids linked together. Variations of proteins are made depending on the order of amino acids. This order is predetermined by the genetic code in the DNA. Proteins don't live forever; their lifespan varies from a few minutes to a few years. Eventually they need to be replicated.

Protein is present in every single cell in our bodies. Proteins have many jobs and work together to perform many functions. Some of the functions of proteins include acting as enzymes, neurotransmitters, and structural components of the cells. Inside each cell there's genetic information called *DNA* that provides instructions for making every type of protein needed by the body. DNA contains the genetic information for how cells will grow, absorb nutrients, act, and the job they will do. When new proteins are needed, *RNA* comes into play.

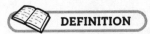 **DEFINITION**

Deoxyribonucleic acid (DNA) is a molecule in your cells that contains the genetic information on how to build and maintain an organism—basically instructions for building a human—you. **Ribonuleic acid (RNA)** is a molecule present in your cells that acts as a messenger to translate the information received from DNA to build proteins.

Inside the center or nucleus of each cell is a system set up like a tiny factory line whose job is to replicate DNA. This system can read the genetic information from DNA, then use this information to make an exact copy of the DNA in the form of messenger RNA. The messenger RNA (mRNA) carries all the instructions needed for making new proteins. Once formed, the mRNA leaves the center of the cell and moves to the outer part of the cell, called the *cytoplasm*.

Located in the cytoplasm is another tiny factory system called *ribosome* whose job is to get all the instructions from the mRNA to make new proteins. Transfer RNA (tRNA) then gathers amino acids and brings them to the ribosome. Ribosomal RNA (rRNA) then uses the amino acids (from the tRNA) and instructions (from the mRNA) to make new proteins. These new proteins exactly match the specifications dictated by the mRNA. This new protein then is released from the ribosome and travels to its predetermined workplace.

Protein serves many functions in the body, including building bones, repairing and replacing damaged cells, and making enzymes, antibodies, and hormones. It also helps maintain bodily fluid levels and pH balance. Additionally, protein aids in the transportation of nutrients and molecules throughout the body.

Due to protein's important role in the body, it has been given the nickname the "ultimate building block" of the body. After all, it makes up 18 to 20 percent of our body weight, with about 40 percent of all the body's protein in muscle.

Now that we've discussed the origin of protein synthesis at the cellular level, let's look at the assembled proteins. Proteins are a sequence of 50 to 20,000 amino acids all linked together. Each sequence is distinct, and one mishap could alter a protein's structure and cause an error to occur, which could translate into a disease or, in other words, a genetic defect.

An amino acid is similar in structure to a carbohydrate, but it contains an amino group (NH_2) and an additional carboxyl group ($COOH$). There are 9 essential amino acids and 11 nonessential amino acids. They're categorized as such because essential amino acids must be obtained from food due to the fact that the body doesn't have the capacity to make them. Nonessential amino acids can be made from other amino acids.

The 9 essential amino acids are tryptophan, threonine, isoleucine, leucine, lysine, methionine, phenylalanine, valine, and histidine. Tryptophan is the most recognizable essential amino acid on the list. It's found in turkey and milk and is conducive to making one feel tired or sleepy.

Key Functions of Essential Amino Acid

Phenylalanine	Aids in the manufacture of brain chemicals used as neurotransmitters
Valine	Aids in muscle growth
Threonine	Maintains the immune system
Tryptophan	Aids in sleep
Isoleucine	Required in the formation of hemoglobin a molecule in blood cells that helps carry oxygen throughout the body
Methionine	Maintains skin
Leucine	Makes hormones
Lysine	Makes enzymes, antibodies, and hormones
Histidine	Involved in the synthesis and production of blood cells

In total, the body needs 20 amino acids, but from the 9 essentials it can synthesize the remaining 11 amino acids, which are alanine, arginine, aspartic acid, asparagine, glutamic acid, glutamine, glycine, proline, serine, cysteine, and tyrosine.

NOTABLE INSIGHT

The hair on your head is made up entirely of dead compacted protein cells called keratin. Just beneath your skin is the hair bulb, which holds the root and anchors the hair. The cells are alive and growing at the root but as they extrude out of the hair follicle through the scalp where you can see it, the cells are no longer living.

The body needs a large pool of amino acids to pick and choose from in order to recombine them to make the type of protein required by the body. It keeps about 100 grams of amino acids available for this purpose. Proteins in the body are constantly being made and broken down and repackaged to the tune of about 300 to 400 grams of body protein per day, which are more grams than you would consume in a day.

Unlike carbohydrates, protein is not stored in the body even though it's an energy nutrient. After the molecule is broken apart, some components are saved or converted to fat, but the majority is released into your urine.

How Proteins Are Broken Down

When you eat protein, the chewing action of the teeth actually begins to break apart some of the long chains of protein. When protein enters the stomach, hydrochloric acid and the enzyme pepsin begin to uncoil the long strands of protein and break them up into smaller strandlike molecules.

Next, these shorter strands move into the small intestine where pancreatic enzymes are released along with additional enzymes, which break the molecules into even smaller particles like single amino acids. These amino acids are transported through the intestinal cells by a carrier protein or by active transport, which requires energy to travel into the mucosal cells. After absorption, they're distributed through the bloodstream to wherever they are needed in the body.

Where to Find Protein

Protein is the building block for more than the human body in this universe. Proteins make up cells in animals and plants alike, albeit in different amounts. The highest amounts per ounce come from animal sources such as meat, poultry, eggs, fish, and shellfish; it's also present in plant foods such as beans, peas, and whole grains, although in lesser amounts. For example, 1 ounce of lean meat contains about 7 grams, whereas 1 ounce of pinto beans contains 2½ grams of protein.

Not all proteins are made equal in nature. When learning about the bioavailability of proteins and their quality in our diet, it's helpful to view humans as animals. Then it makes sense that the proteins found in other animals such as beef and chicken are more like the proteins in our bodies. The proteins in plants are less similar. This means that animal protein is more bioavailable, or easier for our bodies to digest and absorb.

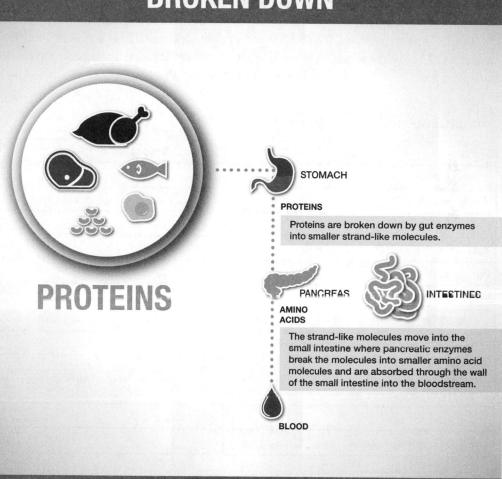

HOW PROTEINS ARE BROKEN DOWN

PROTEINS

STOMACH

PROTEINS

Proteins are broken down by gut enzymes into smaller strand-like molecules.

PANCREAS 　　INTESTINES

AMINO ACIDS

The strand-like molecules move into the small intestine where pancreatic enzymes break the molecules into smaller amino acid molecules and are absorbed through the wall of the small intestine into the bloodstream.

BLOOD

 FOODIE FACTOID

Some proteins take longer to digest than others. For example, whey protein found in dairy can be digested in 1½ hours, whereas the protein in a steak may take 24 to 72 hours. A factor in the protein absorption rate is the nutrients it's accompanied by. An increase in fat or fiber will delay the time it takes for proteins to reach cells in your body. This makes sense in the steak example and is why whey protein shakes are popular among fitness enthusiasts. The protein is extracted from milk and has little to no fat, which allows the protein to be more quickly digested and absorbed and to reach the muscle tissue faster.

Animal-Based Protein

Proteins present in animal foods and animal byproducts contain all of the essential amino acids your body needs, and are considered to be high-quality proteins. However, along with some of those high-protein foods come a higher amount of fat and cholesterol that your body does not benefit from, such as fatty cuts of meat and cholesterol. There are plenty of lean meats, fish, and low-fat options available. The leanest and most tender cuts of beef and pork come from the tenderloin. These have about 1-1½ grams of fat per ounce. Shellfish such as shrimp are also low in fat, and 1 ounce of shrimp contains less than 0.1 gram of fat.

Animal Sources of Protein

Source	Protein in grams
3 oz. beef fillet	18.9
3 oz. ground bison	20.2
3 oz. pork tenderloin	17.7
3 oz. lamb chops	13.8
3 oz. turkey breast	25.5
3 oz. chicken breast	26.4
3 oz. wild salmon fillet	18.0
3 oz. cod fish	19.4
3 oz. bluefin tuna	25.5
3 oz. shrimp	17.8
3 oz. scrambled eggs	13.0
3 oz. 1% fat cottage cheese	10.5

It's easy to meet your protein needs with animal-based protein foods. Most people exceed their needs daily.

 FOODIE FACTOID

Collagen is a protein that forms connective tissues. It's used to make gelatin-type desserts and also used to make marshmallows.

Plant-Based Protein

The majority of plant-based proteins contain limited amounts of the essential amino acids, or they're present in very low amounts to meet your body's requirements for protein synthesis. The exceptions to this are soybeans, quinoa, and spinach, which are considered to be complete protein foods, meaning they contain all nine essential amino acids.

In order for the body to use all the amino acids from noncomplete protein foods, it must combine them with other foods to create complementary proteins. For example, rice and beans are a staple combination in many cultures around the world. They might not have known it under these terms, but ancient civilizations discovered combining rice and beans resulted in healthier people. The limiting amino acid in rice is lysine, which means it's the essential amino acid not present in rice. Beans and legumes contain this amino acid, but they lack methionine. Rice contains plenty of methionine. By combining the two foods, you have a complete protein with all essential amino acids necessary for good health. Complementary proteins don't have to be consumed at the same meal as long as they're eaten during the course of the day.

The following chart shows vegetarian sources of proteins.

Vegetarian Foods High in Protein

Source	Protein in grams
1 cup black beans	15.2
1 cup amaranth	9.4
1 cup lentils	18.0
1 cup chickpeas	14.5
1 cup wild rice	7.0
1 cup buckwheat	5.7
3 tsp. hemp seed	9.0
1 artichoke	3.5
1 cup arugula	5.2
1 cup brown rice	4.5
1 cup brussels sprouts	4.0
¼ cup pecans	5.0
¼ cup almonds	8.0
1 cup asparagus	4.3
½ cup *tempeh*	15.4

Meeting your daily protein requirements can be easily attainable using vegetarian plant-based foods.

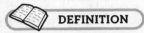 **DEFINITION**

Tempeh is a soy product made from fermented soybeans with the addition of a mold (*Rhizopus oligosporus*) and formed into a shape. It has a firm and chewy texture with a slightly nutty taste.

How Much Do I Need?

The Recommended Dietary Allowance (RDA) for protein ranges from 0.8 grams of protein per kilogram (kg) of body weight to 1.3 grams/kg per day depending on your age, sex, and whether you're pregnant or breastfeeding. The acceptable macronutrient distribution range (AMDR) for protein is 10 to 35 percent of your total calories. Most people require about 0.8 grams of protein per kilogram of body weight per day.

Calculate your protein needs by first converting your body weight from pounds to kilograms (1 pound = 2.2 kilograms). Next multiply your weight in kg × 0.8 grams protein. Let's look at an example:

> 176-pound woman
>
> 176 pounds/2.2 = 80 kilograms
>
> 80 kilograms × 0.8 grams protein = 64 grams protein per day

Pregnant and nursing mothers need more protein to support the growth of a baby as well as additional protein to produce milk. It's recommended that they consume between 10 and 20 grams more daily.

Athletes need more protein as well: about 1.4 to 1.8g/kg/day for strength training and 1.2 to 1.4g/kg/day for endurance runners. Overall, most athletes need about 1.0 to 1.8g/kg/day.

What If I Can't Get Enough?

The average American diet provides well over the recommended daily intake. According to the 2011-2012 National Health and Nutrition Examination Survey, males aged 20-49 average protein intake was 102-104 grams per day and women aged 20-49, 66-72 grams. Protein deficiencies are almost exclusive to developing countries.

When children don't get enough protein in their diet, it's referred to as Protein Energy Malnutrition (PEM), meaning there are either not enough calories or protein to support proper growth and overall bodily functions. Two of the most common PEM conditions are marasmus and kwashiorkor.

Marasmus is a lack of protein and calories in which the infants and small children affected are bony in appearance. Kwashiorkor is a condition resulting from a lack of protein, although calorie levels might be sufficient. This happens when an older child has a high-carbohydrate diet and consumes enough calories throughout the day, but is insufficient in protein. This child has a distended belly from water retention, misleading some people to believe the affected child is full of food or overweight. Since protein plays a role in regulating bodily fluid levels and pH, a child with kwashiorkor has temporarily lost the ability to complete this function successfully.

Although these two PEM conditions exist mostly in developing countries, first-world countries such as the United States are not exempt. Eating disorders such as bulimia, anorexia, and even overeating could be the cause for mild to severe protein deficiencies.

When a person is experiencing a protein deficiency in the diet, the body will begin using the protein in muscles by tearing them down and converting existing proteins to the particular kind that the body is in need of to function. Many factors effect protein needs: stress levels, injuries, increase/decrease in activity level, or breastfeeding, for example.

NOTABLE INSIGHT

Amino acid supplementation is not recommended as it can disrupt your body's normal processes, and leads to an abnormal demand for some amino acids while creating a deficiency for others.

Protein supplements are one method of including more protein in the diet, and there are many available in the marketplace, especially in the form of powders to make protein shakes. There are also protein bars and nutritional ready-to-drink shakes. Animal-based protein powder is made from whey (dairy protein), while vegetarian protein powders are made from ingredients such as soy, brown rice, peas, and artichokes. Most mix easily with water, milk, or milk alternatives such as rice milk and soymilk. Athletes may benefit from supplementing their diets with protein powders for fast digestibility. It's also a good solution for some elderly and the disabled, who are unable or less likely to cook and eat a balanced diet due to mobility or chewing issues.

Is More Protein Better?

Eating more protein than your body needs typically won't harm you if you're in good health. Your body will break down the protein and use whatever it needs, then dispose of the excess and waste byproducts in your urine. However, you may need to consume a little more water to aid in this process.

Many untrained athletes believe that more protein is better because protein helps build muscle. While this is true, eating more won't build more muscle. When a muscle is stressed by lifting weights, it causes small tears in the muscle fibers. The body will use its sources of amino acids to rebuild and repair the protein tears in the muscle, and thus build more muscle.

Some studies have suggested there's a link between high-protein diets and chronic diseases such as heart disease, cancer, and osteoporosis, although research on this topic is limited. In some instances, overconsumption of protein could cause serious problems such as undiagnosed kidney disease, in which case it would place extra stress on the kidneys.

Errors in Protein Metabolism

A rare inherited disorder called phenylketonuria (PKU) occurs when a person has a defect in a gene that helps make the enzyme required to break down phenylalanine. The inability to digest this amino acid leads to a buildup in the body, which causes brain damage along with damage to the central nervous system.

All newborns in the United States are tested for PKU disease. Symptoms can be mild or severe and include delayed development, psychiatric disorders, neurological disorders, and being born with a small head.

Treatment includes following a diet that's low in phenylalanine, along with the addition of vitamin and mineral supplements. Phenylalanine is found in milk, eggs, and other foods. The artificial sweetener aspartame also contains phenylalanine and should be avoided. It's imperative that the diet be strictly followed, as PKU can cause brain damage in the first year of life.

High-Protein Recipe

The following recipe is a great source of high protein. Protein is an indispensable nutrient. Its functions are numerous throughout the body, and it really is the ultimate building block for the body and for good health.

Buffalo Chicken Stuffed Mushrooms

This is a great game-time appetizer with a spicy kick to share with a crowd.

Yield:	Prep Time:	Cook Time:	Serving Size:
24 Servings	25 minutes	15 minutes	1 piece

Each serving has:			
45 calories	1.5g total fat	0g saturated fat	4g protein
4g carbohydrate	0g fiber	10mg cholesterol	115mg sodium

16 oz. baby bella mushrooms

2 TB. olive oil

¼ tsp. kosher salt

⅛ tsp. ground black pepper

12 oz. chicken breast, roughly chopped

¼ cup buffalo sauce

2 cloves garlic

⅔ cup Panko (Japanese bread crumbs)

Sauce

¼ cup light sour cream

2 tsp. buffalo sauce

1. Preheat oven to 400°F.

2. Quickly rinse mushrooms and let drain. Make certain the mushrooms are fairly dry and remove any excess water by patting down with a paper towel.

3. Gently remove stems from the mushroom caps and place the stems into a food processor fitted with a chopping blade. Set aside.

4. Place the caps into a medium-size mixing bowl. Drizzle olive oil over the mushroom caps and add salt and pepper. Toss gently until well coated.

5. Place mushroom caps onto a greased sheet pan.

6. Add to the food processor chicken breast, ¼ cup buffalo sauce, garlic, and Panko. Pulse about 45 seconds or until well combined.

7. Spoon a heaping teaspoon of the chicken mixture into each mushroom cap and place onto sheet pan. Repeat until all caps are stuffed.

8. Bake for about 15 minutes.

9. Combine sour cream and 2 teaspoons buffalo sauce in a small bowl. Mix well. Dollop each mushroom cap with sauce. Serve warm.

The Least You Need to Know

- Protein is found in both plant and animal products.
- There are 9 essential amino acids and 11 nonessential amino acids used as the building blocks of protein by your body.
- Protein works as the body's repair kit.
- Complementary proteins don't need to be consumed at the same time to provide benefits, just over the course of the day.

Fats and Cholesterol

Fats are essential to a healthy diet but can also be detrimental to your health. Getting the right type and in the correct amounts is important for good health. The body is capable of synthesizing most fats from the foods you eat. However, there are two fats that must be consumed through your diet because your body cannot make them: omega-3 and omega-6 fatty acids.

Fats are involved in many functions, such as the absorption of fat-soluble vitamins, insulating your organs, providing your body with energy, and being a part of your cell membranes. Fat is also a flavor carrier and an energy nutrient, which provides 9 calories per gram.

Although fats are an important part of a healthy diet, eating too much of the wrong types can increase your risk of cardiovascular disease and shorten your lifespan.

In This Chapter

- Identifying sources of good and bad fats in foods
- Why is fat essential in your diet?
- How to increase good cholesterol levels
- Do your cholesterol numbers put you at risk?

The Many Types of Fats

The three main categories of fat are unsaturated, saturated, and trans fat. Unsaturated fatty acids can be either monounsaturated or polyunsaturated. The polyunsaturated group contains fats referred to as omega-3s and omega-6s, which are considered essential fatty acids. Saturated fats and trans fats are solid at room temperature. However, they're most commonly found in processed foods.

All fats are made up of carbon and hydrogen atoms with an attached alcohol group. These chains of organic fatty acids are hydrophobic, which means they are not soluble in water.

We're going to take a look at each type of fat, its chemical structure, and where to find it as well as its effect on the body and impact on health.

FOODIE FACTOID

Emulsions are a combination of two liquids that don't normally mix together, like fat and water. Examples of emulsions in common foods are mayonnaise, milk, cream, vinaigrettes, and Hollandaise sauce.

How Fats Are Broken Down

Fats don't readily mix with water, so they cluster together as they move through the digestive system. To break down the fat, bile is released from the gallbladder into the digestive tract. The bile salts in the bile emulsify the fat. Emulsification refers to breaking the large fat clusters of molecules into smaller ones. When the fat is in smaller particles, it's easier for pancreatic lipase, the fat-digesting enzyme, to break it down for digestion. The lipase breaks the fat into free fatty acids and monoglycerides, which are easier for the body to absorb.

Once absorbed, the free fatty acids and monoglycerides are resynthesized into triglycerides inside the epithelial cells of the small intestine. Proteins then coat the triglycerides to form chylomicrons. The protein coating gives the chylomicrons their water-soluble coat and allows them to travel outside of the cell. The chylomicrons leave the epithelial cells and enter the lymphatic capillaries, which allows for their absorption directly into the bloodstream. They circulate in the bloodstream to carry cholesterol and fatty acids to cells throughout the body.

NOTABLE INSIGHT

All fatty acids are not needed immediately for energy use, so the remainder are bound into triglycerides and stored in fat cells. These fat cells have unlimited capacity, and the body is great at storing fat.

Saturated Fat

A saturated fat is a type of fat that is solid at room temperature. "Saturated" refers to its chemical structure being made up of fatty acids heavily laden with hydrogen atoms, which allows for no double bonds between carbon molecules. The hydrogen atoms make the long fatty acid chain more stable because it's difficult for other molecules to knock off a hydrogen atom and cause oxidation. Oxidation makes the fat go rancid.

Health experts agree that saturated fat should only be consumed in limited amounts, as this type of fat can clog arteries. The Dietary Guidelines for Americans recommend consuming no more than 10 percent of calories from saturated fats. This equates to about 22 grams of fat in a 2,000-calorie diet.

Saturated fats come mainly from animal sources of food that include full-fat dairy products (butter and cheese), lard, the fatty portion on the outside of meats as well as the marbling within, and poultry with skin.

Trans Fats

There are two types of trans fat: artificial (made in a lab) and naturally occurring in nature. The primary focus is on the detrimental effects associated with consumption of artificial trans fat. Naturally occurring trans fats like those found in beef, lamb, and butterfat are insignificant sources and very little research has been performed with these types of trans fats in relation to their impact on health.

Trans fats in nature have what is called a "cis" configuration or bend in the molecule. The chemical structure of an artificial trans fat is in a "trans" configuration, which makes its shape straight. It doesn't occur in nature. This shape makes the artificial trans fat very stable and strong. To make trans fats in the lab, liquid oil is heated under pressure and exposed to hydrogen gas and a catalyst. This process is called hydrogenation. The oil is now transformed into a solid and can be used many times without spoilage. It also makes processed foods that contain it less likely to spoil and increases their flavor stability. That's why processed foods contain trans fat. Oil is a very expensive ingredient, and it makes sense why food manufacturers and the restaurant industry would benefit from its use.

In 2002, the National Academy of Sciences recommended that trans fats be eliminated from American diets due to their detrimental effect on health. One study reported that for every 2 percent of trans fat calories in the diet, there was a 23 percent increased risk of cardiovascular disease. Consumption of trans fats has been shown in studies to increase inflammation, insulin resistance, and risk of type 2 diabetes.

Trans fat is often seen in processed foods. However, the Food and Drug Administration (FDA) ruled in June of 2015 that artificial trans fats are to be eliminated from all products over the next 3 years. Food manufacturers can still petition the FDA for certain uses though. The mention of the word "hydrogenated" in the ingredients on the nutrition facts label is usually a sure sign that the food contains trans fat. Food manufacturers are allowed to label food as having 0 grams of trans fat if the food contains less than 0.5 grams of trans fat. For example, some foods will have "partially hydrogenated oil" listed on the food label. Hydrogenation should be a red flag that the product contains trans fats.

 FOODIE FACTOID

Food manufacturers strive to find the perfect levels of ingredients, such as fat, in their food products to optimize palatability. This is called a bliss point, and it's how they get consumers to crave and keep purchasing their products.

Trans fats are most commonly found in shortening, margarine, creamers, crackers, cookies, packaged baked goods, deep-fried foods (french fries, doughnuts, and chicken), and snack foods (chips and microwave popcorn).

Monounsaturated Fats

Monounsaturated fats are liquid at room temperature and will solidify when refrigerated. Their chemical structure has one unsaturated bond in the fatty acid, making the molecule more susceptible to oxidation.

Even though monounsaturated fats are considered heart healthy, they're still fats. The Dietary Guidelines for Americans recommend that Americans consume no more than 10 to 15 percent of their daily calories from monounsaturated fats like olive oil. This is equivalent to 22 to 33 grams per day. One tablespoon of olive oil provides 14 grams of fat.

The health benefits of monounsaturated fats are that they lower LDL (bad) cholesterol levels without adversely affecting your HDL (good) cholesterol levels. Some research has shown that these fats may aid in maintaining blood sugar levels and help improve the function of your blood vessels.

Food sources richest in monounsaturated fats are macadamia nut oil, avocado oil, olive oil, canola oil, macadamia nuts, almonds, cashews, and pecans.

Polyunsaturated Fats

Polyunsaturated fats are essential fatty acids that are necessary for your health. However, your body cannot make them, so you must get them from your food. They're also considered heart healthy. Their chemical structure contains two or more unsaturated bonds in the fatty acid chain, which makes the molecule more susceptible to oxidation and spoilage.

Polyunsaturated fats are further divided into what's called omega-3s and omega-6s, which refers to the position of the double bond in the molecule. Omega-3s and omega-6s like those found in olive and safflower oils are essential to your health. The Dietary Guidelines for Americans recommend that Americans consume no more than 10 percent of their calories from polyunsaturated fats.

The ratio of omega-6s to omega-3s in your diet can influence your risk for chronic diseases. A ratio as close to 1:1 as possible is optimal for health. However, in Western diets the ratio tends to be high in most individuals. Today, the average ratio is upwards of 10:1 and can often be as high as 30:1. Excess omega-6s compete with omega-3s, and thus impact their health benefits. A ratio that's too high can have a negative affect on the body by increasing the risk for cardiovascular disease, cancer, and inflammatory disease.

The health benefits of polyunsaturated fats are that they lower LDL (bad) cholesterol levels. The omega-3s and omega-6s have a variety of specific functions that are beneficial to the body, including maintaining a healthy nervous system and brain function.

Omega-3s

Omega-3s are important for metabolism. These fats are most commonly found in fatty fishes such as salmon, mackerel, tuna, herring, sardines, anchovies, and trout.

Omega-3s benefit the body by reducing triglycerides, controlling irregular heartbeat, slowing plaque buildup, and lowering your blood pressure. Research shows that omega-3s also improve cardiac and vascular hemodynamics, or blood flow.

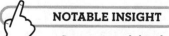

NOTABLE INSIGHT

Some research has found lower levels of depression in cultures that consume high amounts of omega-3s.

Omega-6s

Omega-6s benefit the body by improving blood sugar control, decreasing risk of diabetes, and lowering blood pressure. However, if they are eaten in excess, they can promote an inflammatory response, prevent cell repair, and eventually lead to disease. Research shows an increased risk of developing inflammatory bowel disease (IBD) with high consumption of omega-6s.

Food sources for omega-6s include safflower oil, walnut oil, sunflower oil, corn oil, and soybean corn oil. You should properly balance your intake of omega-6s with your intake of omega-3s.

Triglycerides

A triglyceride is a type of fat. Its chemical structure is made up of three fatty acids attached to a glycerol molecule. Fats from foods you eat and those made by your body don't freely circulate in your blood. They're packaged up into a triglyceride molecule, which typically contains a variety of fatty acids. A triglyceride is the primary storage form of fats in your body. Your body will gather any excess calories from the diet and package them into a triglyceride in order to store it inside your fat cells. An excess consumption of simple carbohydrates like sugary candies or even alcohol can easily increase triglyceride levels. Triglycerides can be released for your body to use as fuel (energy reserves), to insulate body temperature, for shock protection, and to aid the body in the metabolism of carbohydrates and protein.

The American Heart Association (AHA) recommends a triglyceride level of 100mg/dL or less. Check out the following listing to determine where your triglyceride levels rate.

Triglyceride blood levels ranges:

- Normal: Less than 150mg/dL

- Borderline high: 150-199mg/dL

- High: 200-400mg/dL

- Very high: 500mg/dL or above

A high level of triglycerides can harden your arteries and increase the risk of heart disease and stroke, along with obesity and metabolic syndrome. Other conditions that can increase triglyceride levels are uncontrolled type 2 diabetes, hypothyroidism, and liver or kidney disease. Some medications can also increase levels.

 FOODIE FACTOID

The suffix -ol is used to denote a derivative representing alcohol. Examples include glycerol, sorbitol, and ethanol.

To help decrease your triglycerides, you can:

- Reduce alcohol intake.

- Manage blood sugars if diabetic.

- Stop smoking.

- Eat fewer fatty foods.

Cholesterol—the Good and the Bad

Cholesterol is so important to your body that it makes all the cholesterol it needs, so technically you would never need to eat any cholesterol-containing foods. Cholesterol is a waxy substance that's present in all the cells in your body. Chemically, cholesterol is made up of a four-ring carbon structure. This shape reduces permeability of cell membranes and acts as a gatekeeper for certain charged molecules like sodium. Cholesterol also participates in forming bile acids, sex hormones like testosterone, adrenal hormones, and vitamin D.

Your liver manufactures cholesterol and makes about 800 to 1,500mg per day. It also recycles about 50 percent of what it produces, which is reabsorbed within the bowel and carried back into the bloodstream.

When the body makes more than it needs and/or receives too much from the diet, the extra cholesterol often affects the arteries that carry blood from your heart to your body. High levels of circulating cholesterol can damage the epithelial lining of your arteries. LDL cholesterol is especially damaging because it's sticky and thickens your blood. As high levels of LDL circulate through your vessels, some of the LDL becomes oxidized by free radicals. Oxidized LDL encourages the accumulation of inflammatory cells in the inner lining of an artery, which attracts white blood cells and promotes their bonding to the damaged area. The site then becomes laden with more cholesterol and lipids, which continues to increase the thickness of the buildup we call *plaque*.

Plaque formation actually begins in the first decade of life. But plaque build-up can eventually occlude an artery, blocking blood flow completely and leading to a heart attack. A piece of plaque can also break off and create an occlusion that can cause a stroke. This hardening of the arteries is called *atherosclerosis*.

Most people are unaware that they have atherosclerosis until middle age when it causes pain on exertion during exercise or walking. As blood flow is restricted, it results in pain in the legs or chest. Atherosclerosis can affect arteries anywhere in the body. The plaque can burst and cause a blood clot, which can travel throughout the body. Atherosclerosis can cause coronary artery disease (CAD), peripheral artery disease (PAD), cerebrovascular disease, or angina.

Coronary artery disease occurs when the arteries that supply your heart with oxygen, blood, and nutrients become diseased or damaged. The main causes of CAD are plaque buildup and inflammation.

Peripheral artery disease is a condition in which your arteries become narrow and restrict blood flow to your limbs. It's most often caused by atherosclerosis.

Cerebrovascular disease is a variety of disorders that affect the brain by restricting blood flow or by bleeding. A blood vessel may rupture or become narrow or blocked by a blood clot.

Additionally, plaque can cause angina, which is a reduction in adequate blood flow that can cause pain in the chest, shoulders, neck, arms, jaw, or back. This chest pain or discomfort mimics indigestion. Less severe angina commonly occurs upon exertion, such as walking, and will last about 5 minutes with rest.

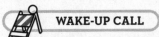 **WAKE-UP CALL**

> The National Institutes of Health (NIH) reports that more than 12.5 million Americans suffer from coronary artery disease and each year it causes 500,000 deaths.

To lower cholesterol levels, eat a low-calorie, low-fat diet and exercise 30 minutes per day. Cholesterol is found in animal food sources including meat, poultry, fish, butter, cheese, and eggs.

High-Density Lipoprotein (HDL)

HDL is considered "good" cholesterol. It's made up of high-density lipoproteins and is a combination of protein, cholesterol, phospholipids, and triglyceride molecules. Protein is found in the greatest percentage at around 50 percent, which is a good thing. HDL's main function is to transport cholesterol back to the liver through the blood. It also removes cholesterol deposited in the walls of blood vessels. Simply stated, HDL keeps your arteries clean and free from blockages.

An HDL cholesterol level of 60mg/dL or greater is considered good. HDL of 40mg/dL is considered low, and you're going to want to try to increase your HDL cholesterol to prevent heart disease.

There are some people who genetically have a high level of HDL so they have added protection, but there are ways you can improve your HDL numbers:

- Replace saturated fat with monounsaturated fats
- Lose weight
- Stop smoking
- Exercise 30 to 60 minutes a day

Low-Density Lipoprotein (LDL)

LDL is considered "bad" cholesterol. It's made up of 50 percent cholesterol, phospholipids, triglycerides, and protein molecules. The function of LDL is to transport cholesterol to the body's cells for use in hormone synthesis. Too much can lead to a build-up of plaque in the arteries, as previously discussed.

Very low density lipoprotein (VLDL) is produced by the liver and released into the bloodstream to supply tissues with triglycerides, which make up about half of VLDL particles. VLDL numbers are often not mentioned during a cholesterol test because there's no direct way to measure them. The number is usually derived as a percent of your triglyceride level. You can lower your VLDL by lowering your triglycerides, losing weight, exercising, and limiting your intake of sugary foods and alcohol.

It's best to keep your intake of high-cholesterol foods at a low or moderate level to help decrease your risk of plaque accumulation. The best way to reduce your LDL cholesterol level is through proper diet and exercise. A good plan is to stop smoking if you do, and to eat foods that are low in fats and high in fiber and omega-3s.

Sometimes diet and exercise aren't enough to bring down LDL levels and your doctor may need to prescribe a cholesterol-lowering medication to your healthy diet and exercise plan.

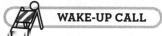

WAKE-UP CALL

An estimated 73.5 million American adults have high LDL levels and less than half receive treatment for it.

Total Cholesterol

The term "total cholesterol" or "total blood (serum) cholesterol" refers to the combination of LDL, VLDL, and HDL cholesterol. It's measured by milligrams of cholesterol per deciliter of blood and is calculated by using the following equation:

HDL + LDL + 20% triglyceride level

A total score of less than 180 mg/dL is considered optimal for your health. When you receive your blood work from your doctor's office, it's already calculated for you. The following are the ranges of cholesterol levels:

Optimal: Below 180 mg/dL

Desireable: Below 200 mg/dL

Borderline high: 200 mg/dL – 239 mg/dL

High: Above 240 mg/dL

The higher your cholesterol level is, the greater your risk of heart disease. People with high cholesterol can also develop a medical condition known as *xanthoma*. It's important to know your numbers. Most physicians recommend cholesterol testing every 5 years or sooner if your lab results are outside of the normal range or if other risk factors are present.

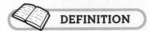 **DEFINITION**

> **Xanthoma** is a skin condition in which cholesterol-rich material is deposited under the surface of the skin. This is most commonly associated with medical conditions that increase blood lipids, such as hyperlipidemia, diabetes, and pancreatitis.

Cholesterol Ratio

Health professionals use the cholesterol ratio to predict your risk of heart disease. To determine your ratio, divide your HDL number by your total cholesterol number. An optimal ratio is less than 3.5:1.0. The greater the cholesterol ratio, the higher your risk of heart disease. This is believed to be a better predictor of heart disease than simply using your LDL or total blood cholesterol levels.

This test accounts for your HDL levels. Two people with the same cholesterol level can have different cholesterol ratios. For example, if you take two people who both have a cholesterol level of 160 but have different HDL levels, they won't have the same ratio. One person has an HDL of 60, so his ratio is 2.7. The other person has an HDL level of 30, so her cholesterol ratio is 5.3. This person would be at an increased risk for developing heart disease.

How to Improve Your Numbers

Changing your diet and lifestyle is the first step toward achieving healthy lipid levels. Research has shown that losing 5 to 10 percent of your total body weight can improve your health. Those who lose weight gradually are more successful at keeping it off and continuing with a healthy lifestyle.

Here are 10 tips to lower your cholesterol and increase your HDL:

1. Aim to lose 5 to 10 percent of your body weight.

2. Work toward a goal of 30 minutes of exercise daily.

3. Decrease or eliminate sources of saturated and trans fats in your diet.

4. Use only healthy fats in your diet.

5. Eat two or more servings of foods rich in omega-3s weekly.

6. Stop smoking.

7. Drink alcohol in moderation.

8. Replace simple carbohydrates with high-fiber foods.

9. Add nuts to your diet.

10. Learn to relax through meditation or yoga.

Discovering Healthy Fats in Foods

Fat is a flavor carrier, but a little will go a long way. If you eat too much fat, as we learned earlier, it will be stored in your body's cells as energy reserves. However, the problem is we never seem to need those extra reserves. We just keep adding more to the stockpile and thus more body weight, which is detrimental to health. Consequently, it's important to choose a healthier type of fat to use in your meals that provides all the health benefits with a taste you can enjoy.

Keep in mind that most Americans consume an unbalanced ratio of essential fatty acids. We have too much omega-6s and too few omega-3s in our diets. So it makes sense that great fats to use in your diet would be ones high in omega-3s.

Top Sources of Heart-Healthy Omega-3 Fats in Foods

Healthier fats can be found in fatty fish, fruits, nuts, oils, and whole grains. The following table includes some of the best sources for omega-3 fats.

Top Sources of Omega-3s

Seafood	Vegetables	Nuts and oils
Salmon	Spinach	Flaxseeds
Anchovies	Broccolini	Chia seeds
Herring	Cauliflower	Walnuts
Mackerel	Arugula	Pecans
Oysters	Butterhead lettuce	Peanuts
Sardines	Turnip greens	Walnut oil
Bluefin tuna	Pinto beans	Canola oil
Sablefish	Kidney beans	Wheat germ oil
Striped bass	Bell peppers	Soybean oil
Rainbow trout		

FOODIE FACTOID

Consuming approximately two 3-ounce servings of fatty fish each week is recommended for their health benefits. However, it's important to limit fish that contain high levels of mercury, including king mackerel, swordfish, shark, and tile fish. Seafood with low levels of mercury but high levels of omega-3s include flounder, herring, salmon, oysters, and canned light tuna.

Healthy Fats Recipe

This recipe highlights the use of healthy fats such as monounsaturated-rich olive oil and omega-3–containing walnuts.

Beet Greens Pesto

Yield:	Prep Time:	Cook Time:	Serving Size:
1 cup	15 minutes	10 minutes	1 TB.

Each serving has:			
60 calories	6g total fat	1g saturated fat	2g protein
1g carbohydrates	0g fiber	0mg cholesterol	95mg sodium

4 cups beet greens, stems removed and roughly chopped

2 garlic cloves

2 TB. lemon juice

1/3 cup Parmesan cheese, freshly grated

1/4 cup walnuts, chopped and toasted

1/4 tsp. kosher salt

1/8 tsp. black pepper

5 TB. extra virgin olive oil

1. Bring a pot of salted water to a boil. Place chopped beet greens in boiling water for 2 minutes. Remove from water and place directly into a bowl of ice water. Let greens stand in ice water for 2 minutes. Drain water and squeeze greens to remove excess water.

2. Add beet greens, garlic, lemon juice, Parmesan cheese, walnuts, salt, and pepper to a food processor fitted with a chopping blade. Turn machine on and slowly drizzle in olive oil while the machine is running for 1 minute, or until mixture is completely combined and smooth. Season with additional salt and pepper to taste.

The Least You Need to Know

- Fat is a flavor carrier and provides satiety in your diet. Eating a little bit of healthy fat may help you eat less later in the day.

- Some people overproduce cholesterol, and when exercise and healthy eating can't lower the numbers, your doctor may prescribe a cholesterol-lowering medication along with a healthy diet and regular exercise.

- Heart-healthy fats can be found in certain types of fish, nuts, and oils, and whole grains.

Vitamins

Vitamins are essential for health. Your body is capable of making some of the 13 vitamins needed for it to function properly, but others must be obtained from the foods you eat.

In this chapter, we'll take a look at the important role of each vitamin and how your body uses them to support normal cell function and growth. We will learn how much you need each day and examine which vitamins can be toxic when taken in high doses, along with the detrimental effects in your body.

In This Chapter

- Distinguishing between water-soluble and fat-soluble vitamins

- The process of vitamin absorption and digestion

- B vitamins and their role in the body

- Getting the right amount of the Recommended Daily Allowance (RDA) for vitamins

- How to avoid vitamin toxicity

What Is a Vitamin?

Vitamins are naturally occurring organic compounds that are required by the body for nutrition and growth. These essential micronutrients must be obtained through diet because the body is unable to produce enough of these compounds on its own.

There are 13 vitamins that are classified as either fat-soluble or water-soluble. Fat-soluble vitamins are A, D, E, and K, and they're stored in the liver or in fatty tissues. The water-soluble vitamins include all of the B vitamins and vitamin C. They're not stored as long in the body, and the excess is usually released through urine. Therefore, water-soluble vitamins need to be obtained from food sources in your diet every day.

How Vitamins Are Broken Down in the Body

Vitamins are broken down by the mechanical chewing action of your teeth. Food is mixed with saliva and enzymes as you chew. The food is swallowed and transferred from the esophagus to the stomach, where it encounters hydrochloric acid and more enzymes, which aid in the release of nutrients.

The fat-soluble vitamins require the addition of bile so they can be emulsified prior to absorption in the small intestine. Water-soluble vitamins don't require bile. Once absorbed in the small intestine, the nutrients are released into your bloodstream. The vitamins are next transported to the liver, where one of three things can happen: they're instantly used by the body, carried to the kidneys to be excreted, or stored in the liver or fatty tissues until the body needs them.

Absorption of vitamins can be disrupted if chronic conditions like alcoholism are present or there's a disease state within the body. Alcoholism could damage the liver, stomach, and intestines, which are all involved in vitamin absorption and digestion. Intestinal diseases such as Crohn's disease, irritable bowel syndrome, or any prolonged inflammation of the digestive tract could also interfere with absorption and digestion of vitamins.

Water-Soluble Vitamins

Water-soluble vitamins can be dissolved in water and are not stored in your body. There are nine water-soluble vitamins, including vitamin C and the B vitamins: thiamin (vitamin B_1), riboflavin (vitamin B_2), niacin (vitamin B_3), pyridoxine (vitamin B_6), folate (folic acid), vitamin B_{12}, biotin, and pantothenic acid.

The B Vitamins

The B vitamins are responsible for a variety of processes in the body, such as aiding in energy production from the macronutrients and in the formation of red blood cells. Some B vitamins also function as *coenzymes*. A deficiency of certain B vitamins can lead to anemia, which causes fatigue and weakness.

B vitamins can be found in proteins like red meat, fish, poultry, eggs, and dairy products. They're also present in dark-green leafy vegetables, and legumes. Let's take a more detailed look at each of these vitamins.

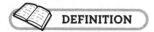 **DEFINITION**

A **coenzyme** is a molecule that needs an enzyme to initiate or create a chemical reaction.

Vitamin B12

Vitamin B12 is responsible for the health of your body's nerve and blood cells. It also helps produce DNA and RNA, which are the genetic material found in all cells. Vitamin B12 also works with folic acid to produce red blood cells and regulate iron in your body. Due to vitamin B12's influence on red blood cells, this vitamin can also aid in prevention of megaloblastic anemia. Megaloblastic anemia is when your body makes blood cells that are very large, structurally abnormal, and immature. This abnormal cell is unable to carry a sufficient amount of oxygen to your body's tissues.

Your body is unable to produce vitamin B12 on its own, so it must be obtained through the diet. Although certain types of bacteria may produce B12 within the body, the amount is not sufficient to guarantee adequate nutrition.

During the digestion of B12 in the stomach, hydrochloric acid will first separate the vitamin from the protein molecule. Next, in order for B12 to survive the harsh acids in the stomach, it must combine with another protein produced by the stomach known as *intrinsic factor*. Once bound with intrinsic factor, it can travel on to the small intestine where the intrinsic factor will be degraded. The B12 is absorbed into the bloodstream and is delivered to the liver for distribution.

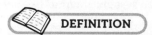 **DEFINITION**

Intrinsic factor is an essential glycoprotein that's produced by the parietal cells within the stomach in order for your body to efficiently absorb vitamin B12. Without intrinsic factor, your body can't recognize B12.

Without intrinsic factor, you can develop a type of vitamin B₁₂ deficiency called *pernicious anemia*. Pernicious anemia will lead to megaloblastic anemia. This form of anemia affects red blood cell production by producing fewer cells that are large and immature when compared to healthy red blood cells. This irregularity impacts the cells' ability to transport oxygen.

Some people don't make enough intrinsic factor or have a chronic condition that destroys it. Digestive tract disorders such as irritable bowel syndrome (IBS) and Crohn's disease will cause your body to stop producing intrinsic factor. If the stomach has been surgically removed due to disease or injury, your body will not be able to produce intrinsic factor. Alcoholism, *H. pyloric* bacterial infections, ulcerative gastritis, Zollinger-Ellison syndrome, gastric bypass surgery, and even age can negatively impact the production of intrinsic factor.

The *Recommended Daily Allowance (RDA)* for vitamin B₁₂ for adults is 2.4 mcg. The following table lists more detailed information for RDAs. There's no known toxicity for B₁₂.

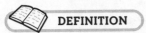

> **DEFINITION**
>
> **Recommended Dietary Allowance (RDA)** is the average daily intake level that meets health requirements for the majority of the population.

Vitamin B₁₂ is found in animal foods, such as meats, poultry, fish, eggs, and dairy. Additionally, vitamin B₁₂ can be found in fortified foods such as cereals.

Vitamin B₆

Vitamin B₆ has three forms: pyridoxal, pyridoxamine, and pyridoxine. Each type can be used to form nonessential amino acids in metabolism. B₆ is involved in hundreds of enzymatic reactions, along with aiding in the body's immune system and cognitive abilities, as well as production and use of glucose.

Vitamin B₆ is digested and absorbed in the jejunum by a process of passive diffusion. Passive diffusion is a way for small molecules to simply diffuse across a membrane.

The RDA for vitamin B₆ for adult males and females age 19 to 50 years old is 1.3mg per day. See the following table for more detailed information.

A deficiency of vitamin B₆ is uncommon but can cause neurological problems, depression, fatigue, microcytic anemia, skin disorders, and a weakened immune system. Vitamin B₆ deficiency can occur when excessive alcohol is consumed, and if you have kidney disease or malabsorption disorders.

The tolerable upper limit (UL) for B₆ for adults is 100mg per day. High intake of B₆ from food or supplements can cause peripheral neuropathy.

Many foods contain vitamin B6. Sources include fortified cereals, meats, poultry, fish, fruit, and starchy vegetables such as peas and potatoes.

RDA for Vitamin B12 and B6

Age	B12 (mcg)	B6 (mg)
Birth-6 months	0.4	0.1 males/0.1 females
Infants 7-12 months	0.5	0.3 males/0.3 females
Children 1-3 years	0.9	0.5 males/0.5 females
Children 4-8 years	1.2	0.6 males/0.6 females
Children 9-13 years	1.8	1.0 males/1.0 females
Teens 14-18	2.4	1.3 males/1.2 females
Adults	2.4	1.3 males/1.3 females
Adults 51 and over	2.4	1.7 males/1.5 females
Pregnant teens and women	2.6	1.9
Breastfeeding teens and women	2.8	2.0

Thiamin, Riboflavin, and Niacin

Thiamin, or vitamin B1, takes part in a variety of chemical reactions in your body. Thiamin's primary function is to assist cells in converting carbohydrates into energy. Thiamin also assists with transmission of nerve signals and the contraction of muscles.

The RDA of thiamin for adult males is 1.2mg and for females 1.1mg per day. For more detailed information, refer to the following table. There's no known toxicity associated with thiamin.

Thiamin deficiency is rare in the United States and is typically associated with alcoholism (Wernicke-Korsakoff syndrome). Symptoms of thiamin deficiency are loss of appetite, weight loss, irregular heart rate, muscle weakness, psychosis, weakness, and nerve damage. Continual thiamin deficiency can lead to a disease called *beriberi*, which can cause cardiovascular and peripheral nervous system damage. In very severe cases, brain damage can occur.

 NOTABLE INSIGHT

Beriberi is caused by a deficiency of B1, and historically it was found in regions where people were dependent on polished rice as a food staple. The polished rice had a longer shelf life, but the process also stripped the thiamin away.

Thiamin can be found in a variety of foods including whole grains, rice, pasta, flour, bread, cereals, beef, pork, eggs, nuts, seeds, legumes, and peas.

Riboflavin, or vitamin B2, is involved in energy metabolism and serves as a coenzyme. These active forms of riboflavin are flavin mononucleotide (FMN) and flavin adenine dinucleotide (FAD). Riboflavin also functions as an antioxidant by protecting the body from free radicals.

The RDA for adult men is 1.3mg per day and for adult women 1.1mg per day. There's no known toxicity associated with thiamin and no tolerable upper limits have been established. Riboflavin deficiency is very rare and is typically seen in conjunction with other vitamin deficiencies.

Riboflavin can be found in eggs, dairy products, lean proteins, legumes, dark-green leafy vegetables, nuts, and fortified breads and cereals. Riboflavin is also very sensitive to light exposure and is easily destroyed if foods are not kept in dark storage areas.

Niacin, or vitamin B3 is also known as nicotinic acid and nicotinamide (niacinamide). Niacin functions as a coenzyme in the body, where it's involved in energy metabolism. It also aids in the synthesis of fatty acids and cholesterol. The body can also make niacin from tryptophan.

The RDA for niacin for adult males is 16mg per day and for females 14mg per day. The tolerable upper limit is for adults 35mg per day. Toxicity symptoms are flushing of the skin, hives, nausea and vomiting, and liver damage.

Niacin deficiency was common in the 1800s and was called *pellagra*, which caused dermatitis, diarrhea, dementia, and eventually death.

Niacin can be found in meats, poultry, fish, eggs, dairy, nuts, and legumes.

RDA for Thiamin, Riboflavin, and Niacin

Age/Gender	Thiamin (mg)	Riboflavin (mg)	Niacin (mg)
0–6 months	0.2	0.3	0.2
7–12 months	0.3	0.4	0.4
Children 1–3	0.5	0.5	0.6
4–8	0.6	0.6	0.8
9–13	0.9	0.9	12
Males 14+	1.2	1.3	16
Females 14–18	1.0	1.0	14
Females 19+	1.1	1.1	14

Biotin, Pantothenic Acid, and Folate

Biotin functions as a coenzyme in the body used in energy metabolism. It's also involved in the production of glucose and synthesis/breakdown of fatty acids.

There's no RDA established for biotin, but the *Adequate Intake (AI)* for adult males is 25 mcg per day and for females 30 mcg. Refer to the following table for more information.

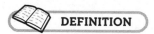 **DEFINITION**

> **Adequate Intake (AI)** is a value used that is an approximation of required nutrient levels when the Recommended Dietary Allowance (RDA) can't be determined.

Deficiency of biotin is rare because your body can recycle it. There's also no known toxicity of biotin.

Biotin can be found in a variety of foods such as egg yolks, liver, fish, and whole grains.

Known as vitamin B_5, pantothenic acid forms part of the structure of coenzyme A, which is found in cells. It participates in chemical reactions involved in the release of energy from macronutrients; the synthesis of lipids; hemoglobin, hormones, and neurotransmitters.

There's no RDA for pantothenic acid, but the AI for adults is 5mg per day. There are no known toxicity levels.

Food sources for pantothenic acid include liver, fish, shellfish, poultry, egg yolks, dairy products, broccoli, legumes, mushrooms, and whole grains. Freezing and canning will reduce its bioavailability.

Folate, folacin, or folic acid is also known as B_9 or its chemical name, pteroylglutamic acid (PGA). It functions as a coenzyme in the body. It also helps convert B_{12} to an active form and aids in synthesis of DNA and new cell formation. It's digested by enzymes and absorbed in the small intestine. Excess folate is secreted into bile by the liver, and then it's returned to the gall bladder for storage.

The RDA for adults is 400mcg per day. The tolerable upper limit is established at 1,000mcg per day. There are no known toxicity levels. However, folate supplementation could mask megaloblastic anemia caused by a B_{12} deficiency. Deficiency of folate can lead to megaloblastic anemia. It can also cause neural tube birth defects such as spina bifida.

> **NOTABLE INSIGHT**
>
> Neural tube defects affect the brain, spine, or spinal cord in a fetus, and occur during the first month of pregnancy. An adequate intake of folic acid prior to pregnancy can prevent most cases.

Folate can be found in a variety of foods like green leafy vegetables, legumes, citrus fruits, and fortified foods such as breads, cereals, pasta, and rice.

AI for Biotin, Pantothenic Acid, and RDA for Folate

Age/Gender	Biotin (mcg) AI	Pantothenic Acid (mg) AI	Folate (mcg) RDA
Birth-6 months	5	1.7	65
7-12 months	6	1.8	80
Children 1-3	8	2	150
Children 4-8	12	3	200
Children 9-13	20	4	300
Males 14+	25	5	400
Females 14–18	30	5	400 600 (pregnant teens)
Females 19+	30	5	400
Pregnant women	30	6	500
Breastfeeding females	35	7	600 (14-18 years) 500 (19 and older)

Vitamin C

Vitamin C is a water-soluble vitamin and is sometimes called ascorbic acid. Its role in the body is to function as an antioxidant, aid in the production of collagen, and support your immune system. As an antioxidant, it works in the body by protecting against free radicals that damage cells. Free radicals are byproducts of normal metabolism, but they also come from outside sources such as pollution, cigarette smoke, and exposure to UV light.

When your body is physically stressed due to the presence of an infection or serious injury, adrenal glands release vitamin C to support immune functions. Vitamin C ensures that the oxidative process involving free radical release runs smoothly.

Vitamin C helps make collagen, which is a fibrous protein used in building bones and teeth. It also helps strengthen veins and capillary walls, along with aiding in wound repair. It supports collagen formation by protecting iron molecules from being oxidized during the formation of collagen. Without vitamin C's action, no protein would be formed and tissue repair, such as in the formation of scars, would never occur.

 FOODIE FACTOID

British sailors were called "limeys" because they carried limes on their voyages to prevent the vitamin C deficiency disease called scurvy.

Deficiency of vitamin C is rare in the United States, as you would have to consume less than 10mg over several weeks to develop scurvy. One orange provides 70mg of vitamin C.

The RDA for vitamin C is provided in the following table. If you're a smoker, add 35mg daily.

RDA for vitamin C

Age	Recommended amount in milligrams (mg)
Birth-6 months	40
Infants 7-12 months	50
Children 1-3 years	15
Children 4-8 years	25
Children 9-13 years	45
Teens 14-18 years (boys)	75
Teens 14-18 years (girls)	65
Adult males	90
Adult females	75
Pregnant teens and women	80 (pregnant teens) 85 (pregnant adult women)
Breastfeeding teens and women	115 (breastfeeding teens) 120 (breastfeeding adult women)

Vitamin C can be found in a variety of fruits and vegetables. We typically look to citrus fruits such as oranges and grapefruits, but bell peppers, broccoli, and tomatoes are also good sources.

The tolerable upper intake limit for Vitamin C for adults is 200mg per day. If you overconsume vitamin C, it can lead to headache, nausea, diarrhea, stomach cramps, fatigue, and hot flashes. However, you would have to take an excess of over 4,000 mg per day.

Fat-Soluble Vitamins

The fat-soluble vitamins are A, D, E, and K. These vitamins provide a variety of functions in the body: keeping your eyes healthy, strengthening your bones, protecting your cells, and clotting blood. Because these vitamins are fat-soluble, they must be emulsified by bile before your body can absorb them. Additionally, many need a protein carrier to travel through the bloodstream. Unlike water-soluble vitamins, fat-soluble vitamins can be stored in the liver and fatty body tissues, which allows your body to release the vitamins on demand. It also means you don't necessarily need to eat foods containing that particular vitamin every day because your body can store it. Unfortunately, with A, D and E, you can reach toxic levels that can be detrimental to your health.

Vitamin A

There are three forms of vitamin A. One type (retinol) is from animal sources and is also referred to as preformed vitamin A. The other two, retinal and retinoic acid (alpha carotene and beta-carotene) are from plant sources and are also known as provitamin A. Vitamin A performs many functions in the body. It helps promote normal vision and the growth of healthy cells, regulates the immune system, and is important for embryo development.

Vitamin A supports your vision by keeping the cornea of the eye healthy. It also helps you see in the dark by aiding in the chemical reaction within the eye that has to do with the absorption of wavelengths of light.

Vitamin A plays an important role when it comes to cellular growth and division in the body. This vitamin aids in protein synthesis and cell differentiation, which means each cell is told what job it will perform, ranging from being a skin cell on the outside of your body to being a mucous cell on the inside of your body lining the GI tract.

Vitamin A is important in the reproductive cycle for men and women. In men, the vitamin helps sperm development. In women, it aids in fetal development.

The RDA for adult males is 900mcg retinol activity equivalents (RAE) per day and for women 700mcg. RAE is a unit of measure and refers to the body's ability to convert provitamin carotenoids into vitamin A. For more detailed information, refer to the table at the end of this section.

 FOODIE FACTOID

Carrots are a good source of beta-carotene. Americans consume just over 10 pounds per person each year.

Deficiencies of vitamin A are rare in the United States. However, it's the leading cause of blindness in developing countries. Deficiency symptoms are corneal drying, which leads to blindness, impaired immunity, and plugged hair follicles that cause white bumps to appear on the skin, referred to as hyperkeratosis.

Since vitamin A can be stored in the body, it's possible to reach toxic levels. The tolerable upper limit for adults 19 and older is 3,000mcg per day. Toxicity can cause birth defects, reduced bone density, blurred vision, vertigo, headaches, and abnormal muscle function.

It's easy to get plenty of vitamin A from foods, such as eggs, liver, spinach, broccoli, vitamin A-fortified dairy products, and orange-colored fruits and vegetables such as apricots, winter squashes, carrots, and sweet potatoes.

Vitamin D

The primary function of vitamin D is to help make strong bones by aiding in the body's ability to absorb calcium. It also supports neurotransmissions and strengthens the immune system.

Vitamin D is also known as calciferol and is technically a hormone. Your body can make vitamin D from exposure to sunlight. A chemical compound of vitamin D is made from cholesterol in your liver. The liver releases this compound, which then travels to the skin and the ultraviolet light from the sun changes the molecule into previtamin D_3, an inactive form. It then travels to the liver where the molecule is changed into 25-hydroxy vitamin D_3, and then moves into the kidneys where it is converted into the active form vitamin D_3 (1,25-dihydroxy vitamin D_3). Therefore, if you receive regular sunlight exposure, there is no need to consume food sources of vitamin D.

Vitamin D helps support bone growth by maintaining a tight control on blood levels of calcium and other minerals such as phosphorus, magnesium, and fluoride. This vitamin can direct the body to absorb more calcium in the GI tract or pull it from the bones. It works in conjunction with the kidneys and other hormones to ensure there's an adequate supply of minerals in the blood.

Recommended intake for adults 19-70 years old is 600IU. Refer to the table at the end of this section for more detailed information.

Vitamin D deficiency disease is rare in the United States. When there are insufficient amounts of vitamin D in the body, the bones don't calcify properly and it causes the leg bones to bow outwards in children. Known as *rickets,* this occurs because the bones are too weak to support the weight of the child, and is why dairy products are fortified with vitamin D. Rickets also causes beaded ribs, which are malformations between the attachment of bone and cartilage.

Additional symptoms are bone pain and low levels of calcium in the blood. In adults a vitamin D deficiency can cause soft bones, a condition called *osteomalacia*. Kidney disease is also a factor that could lead to a vitamin D deficiency since it's so closely tied to the production of vitamin D.

Excess consumption of vitamin D can lead to toxicity. It will cause too much calcium to be released into the blood where it can harden blood vessels and arteries. It can also cause the formation of kidney stones.

 NOTABLE INSIGHT

To get your daily dose of vitamin D from the sun, you need 15 minutes of exposure.

Sources of vitamin D in the diet are fortified-food products, such as dairy, along with egg yolks, liver, fatty fish, veal, and beef.

Vitamin E

Vitamin E is also known as tocopherol. Scientists actually discovered multiple forms of tocopherol, but only one is active in the body. Its primary function is to work as an antioxidant to protect cells from damage by free radicals. Vitamin E also prevents oxidation of LDL cholesterol, and it aids in the formation of red blood cells and maintains stores of vitamins A, K, iron, and selenium.

Recommended vitamin E intake for in adults is 15mg. Refer to the table at the end of this section for more detailed information.

Vitamin E deficiency is rare and typically linked to a fat malabsorption disease. Without adequate amounts of vitamin E, nerve and muscle damage can occur, including muscle weakness and loss of feeling in the extremities, along with impaired vision and an immune system.

Consumption of excess amounts of vitamin E from dietary sources is not toxic. However, additional intake from supplements may affect the body's ability to clot blood. The tolerable upper limit is 1,000mg per day.

Vitamin E can be found in vegetable oils, nuts, spinach, broccoli, and fortified foods like breakfast cereals and margarine.

Vitamin K

There are actually many compounds that make up what we refer to as Vitamin K. Phylloguinone is a natural form of vitamin K found in green plants, and menaquinones are a natural form made by bacteria. Menadione is a synthetic form of vitamin K that can be converted by enzymes to an active form in the body.

Vitamin K's function in the body is to assist in the role of blood clotting. It also aids in bone formation by helping calcium bind to the protein matrix in the structure of bones.

Recommended daily intake for adult males is 120mcg and for females 90mcg. Refer to the table at the end of this section for more detailed information.

Deficiency of vitamin K can lead to hemorrhaging, but it's rare. Newborn babies are dosed with vitamin K because vitamin K doesn't pass through the placenta, and they also don't have sufficient gut bacteria to produce it on their own.

There's no known toxicity associated with natural forms of vitamin K and thus the Food and Nutrition Board of the Institute of Medicine has established no tolerable upper limits. However, large amounts of the synthetic form could cause liver damage.

 WAKE-UP CALL

Do not consume foods high in vitamin K if you're on a blood thinner like Coumadin. Vitamin K can adversely interact with the medication.

Food sources of vitamin K are leafy greens, broccoli, cauliflower, liver, fermented dairy and soy products, wheat bran, and green tea.

RDA for vitamins A and E, AIs for vitamins D and K

Age/Gender	Vitamin A (mcg) RAE	Vitamin E (mg)	Vitamin D (mcg)	Vitamin K (mcg)
Birth-5 months	400	4	5	2
5-12 months	500	5	5	2.5
Children 1-3	300	6	5	30
Children 4-8	400	7	5	55
Males 9-13	600	11	5	60
Males 14-18	600	11	5	75
Males 19-30	900	15	5	120
Males 31-50	900	15	5	120
Males 51-70	900	15	10	120
Males 71 & Up	900	15	15	120
Females 9-13	900	11	5	60

continues

RDA for vitamins A and E, AIs for vitamins D and K   (continued)

Age/Gender	Vitamin A (mcg) RAE	Vitamin E (mg)	Vitamin D (mcg)	Vitamin K (mcg)
Females 14-18	600	15	5	75
Females 19-30	700	15	5	90
Females 31-50	700	15	5	90
Females 51-70	700	15	10	90
Females 71 & Up	700	15	15	90
Pregnant Women >18	750	15	5	75
19-30	770	15	5	90
31-50	770	15	5	90
Breastfeeding >18	1,200	19	5	75
19-30	1,300	19	5	90
31-50	1,300	19	5	90

The Least You Need to Know

- Fat-soluble vitamins are stored in the body's tissues. It's best not to take excessive amounts in supplement form.
- Water-soluble vitamins aren't stored in the body and need to be consumed daily in your diet.
- Inadequate intake of B_6 and B_{12} can lead to anemia, which causes fatigue and weakness.

CHAPTER 10

Minerals

Your body needs minerals in various amounts for good health. Some minerals help regulate fluid balance, strengthen bones, aid in muscle movement, and communication between cells. Your body can also store some minerals, too, unlike water-soluble vitamins.

In this chapter, we'll take a look at the role of minerals and how your body uses them along with how much you need every day. You'll learn what happens when you don't get a sufficient amount of the required minerals and the effects on your body. You'll also discover the best food sources for them.

In This Chapter

- How the body uses minerals for support and growth
- The digestion and absorption of minerals
- Best food sources for the right amount of minerals in your diet
- What happens when you don't get enough?
- Can you get too many minerals in your diet?

What Is a Mineral?

Minerals are inorganic elements, meaning they do not contain carbon and occur naturally in soil and water. Plants absorb minerals through their roots, and you obtain the minerals when you eat the plant or the animal that consumed the plant. Minerals are very stable compounds and water-soluble. They're not adversely affected by stomach acid, heat, exposure to oxygen, or ultraviolet light.

Minerals are divided into two groups: major minerals and trace minerals. The major minerals are those required in amounts more than 100mg per day, and trace minerals are required in amounts less than 20mg per day. Calcium is an example of a major mineral and iron is a trace mineral. In this chapter, we'll take a detailed look at the many ways your body uses these minerals.

How Minerals Are Broken Down in the Body

Minerals are charged molecules and are unable to travel freely through the digestive tract without the aid of a protein molecule carrier so they can be absorbed. Minerals also compete with one another in the GI tract. If you overload your system with an abundance of calcium, it may use all the available protein carriers in the GI tract and prevent other minerals from being absorbed in the correct proportions.

Vitamins can also impact mineral absorption. Vitamin C enhances iron absorption from plant food sources. Vitamin D increases the absorption of calcium, phosphorus, and magnesium. Your body has the ability to increase or decrease the absorption rates of minerals based on how much of a particular mineral it has stored away. For example, if you need more calcium, your body will absorb more from the food you eat. If the body's stores of calcium are high, it will absorb less calcium from a meal and utilize what is stored.

There are also some compounds that block the absorption of minerals. For example, oxalates are found in some vegetables such as spinach, and they prevent calcium from being absorbed by the body. Other examples include the polyphenols in tea and phytates in grains.

Major Minerals

The major minerals are calcium, magnesium, sodium, phosphorus, sulfate, potassium, sodium, and chloride. The primary role of these minerals in the body is to build bones and blood cells, support immune health, maintain *fluid balance*, and activate enzymes.

Some minerals are referred to as *electrolytes*, which aid in the maintenance of your body's fluid balance inside and outside of the cells. Electrolytes are positively and negatively charged molecules. Protein is also involved in the body's fluid balance, as discussed in Chapter 7.

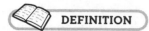 **DEFINITION**

Fluid balance occurs when the amount of fluid taken in equals the amount lost from the body. **Electrolytes** are minerals that help the body retain or excrete fluids when necessary.

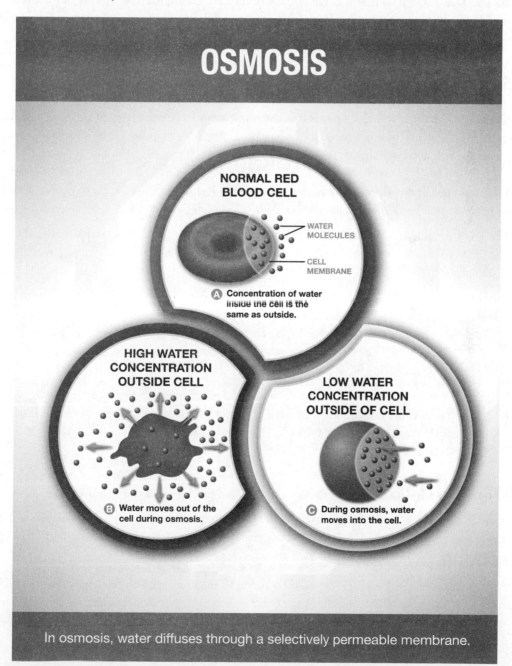

OSMOSIS

NORMAL RED BLOOD CELL

WATER MOLECULES

CELL MEMBRANE

Ⓐ Concentration of water inside the cell is the same as outside.

HIGH WATER CONCENTRATION OUTSIDE CELL

Ⓑ Water moves out of the cell during osmosis.

LOW WATER CONCENTRATION OUTSIDE OF CELL

Ⓒ During osmosis, water moves into the cell.

In osmosis, water diffuses through a selectively permeable membrane.

Water follows electrolytes by moving to wherever there's a higher electrolyte concentration. Sodium and chloride are on the outside of the cell and other electrolytes reside on the inside of the cell. A cell only allows certain molecules to pass freely across its membrane, and water is one of these molecules. If there's an elevated amount of sodium outside the cell than electrolytes inside the cell, water will pass freely to the outside of the cell to equalize the concentration inside and outside the cell. The ratio of solids to liquids is therefore changed. This process is called *osmosis*.

Let's take a look at each mineral and its role in your body.

Calcium

Calcium is the most abundant mineral in the body, with 99 percent located in the bones and teeth. We know calcium is needed for strong bones, but it's also involved in muscle movement, neurotransmissions to help the cells communicate, and the movement of blood throughout the body. Additionally, it works with a variety of hormones and enzymes. Most people fall short when it comes to an adequate intake (AI) of calcium. Postmenopausal women, people with lactose intolerance, and vegans are at a higher risk for calcium deficiency.

The RDA for calcium in adults 19 to 50 years old is 1,000mg per day. To enhance the absorption of supplements, it's best to divide the amount into two 500mg doses. Women over 50 need 1,200mg per day.

Calcium intake is critical during periods of peak bone mass formation. From birth to age 20 is the first phase, in which about 90 percent of bone mass is acquired. Bone mass can continue to grow until age 30. The calcium laid down during these periods will affect your bone density rate as you age. After age 30, bone density begins a steady decline and a low intake of calcium early on can lead to osteomalacia and osteoporosis.

Calcium in too high amounts can interfere with the absorption of other minerals such as iron and zinc. It will also cause constipation. In some adults, it can increase the formation of kidney stones. The upper limit for calcium for adults age 19 to 50 is 2,500mg per day and for adults 51 and older 2,000mg per day.

The best sources of calcium in the diet are found in dairy products. However, broccoli, kale, cabbage, fish with soft bones (sardines), and fortified products like breakfast cereals, dairy alternatives, and tofu can also provide calcium.

Phosphorus

Phosphorus is the second most abundant mineral in the body with the majority stored in bones and teeth. The role of phosphorus in the body is to act as a buffer in regulating acid-base balance and aid in energy metabolism and cell communication. It's also part of DNA, RNA, and the structure of some lipids.

The RDA for phosphorus for adults is 700mg per day. Deficiencies of phosphorus would be a rare occurrence as it's found in most food sources, with liver and dairy being the highest.

The tolerable UL of phosphorus for adults is 4,000mg per day. However, hyperphosphatemia is more commonly seen in those with abnormal kidney function.

When considering food sources of phosphorus, it's important to note that only about 50 percent of phosphorus in beans, peas, cereals, and nuts are absorbable due to phosphorus being bound by phytates. Eggs, milk, salmon, beef, turkey, and chicken are all excellent sources.

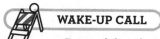

WAKE-UP CALL

Research has shown that an increase in blood phosphorus levels can be an indicator for high levels of calcification in the coronary arteries.

Sulfate

Sulfate helps form the shapes of proteins, especially in hair, nails, and skin. Sulfate is the only mineral that does not have an RDA. The reasoning behind this is that sulfate can be found in a variety of foods and animal proteins. Additionally, sulfate is provided in the body by the amino acids methionine and cysteine.

Therefore, a sulfate deficiency is unlikely to occur unless there was an insufficient protein intake in the diet. Toxicity is also unlikely to occur. Sulfate is present in all protein-containing foods like eggs, meats, fish, poultry, legumes, and nuts.

Potassium

Potassium aids in the maintenance of acid-base balance, electrical activity of the heart, building proteins, and carbohydrate metabolism. Potassium is a positively charged ion. Potassium can decrease calcium excretion when the body needs more calcium present. When the body has too much circulating potassium, it's excreted in urine. The hormone aldosterone regulates this mechanism.

The RDA for potassium for adults 19 and older is 4.7 grams per day.

A deficiency of potassium is called *hypokalemia*. It causes muscle weakness, abnormal heart rhythms, and increased blood pressure. Potassium can also be toxic in high levels, and this is called *hyperkalemia*. High levels of potassium could lead to a dangerous disruption of heart rhythms. Typical causes of hyperkalemia are kidney disease, medications, and infections.

A variety of foods contain potassium, including meats, fish, dairy, soy products, fruits, and vegetables.

Sodium

Sodium is part of a molecule bound with chlorine that makes up table salt (sodium chloride). Sodium has many important functions, such as regulation of fluid balance, maintaining blood pressure, and aiding in nerve and muscle function.

The intake of sodium for Americans is quite high; the average U.S. daily intake ranges from 4 to 6 grams. The RDA for adults is 2,300mg or 1,500mg if you have hypertension. One teaspoon of salt contains about 2,300mg of sodium. However, most people don't exceed sodium recommendations from the salt they add to foods when cooking. Excess sodium comes from processed foods and meals eaten away from home.

Sodium deficiency can lead to low sodium levels in the blood, known as *hyponatremia*, which can cause headaches, muscle weakness, spasms, or cramps, along with nausea and vomiting. It can also lead to seizures or even coma. Diseases such as kidney disease and congestive heart failure can also cause hyponatremia. Other causes include certain medications, alteration in hormone levels, and drinking too much water. Acute illnesses that cause excessive diarrhea and vomiting can lead to low sodium levels as well.

Hypernatremia is an excess of sodium in the blood, usually caused by a deficit of water in the body. It typically occurs in elderly individuals who are dependent on others for food and fluid needs. Intravenous feeding solutions or excessive fluid loss due to diarrhea and vomiting can lead to hypernatremia.

There's no toxicity level associated with sodium. Sodium is naturally present in fruits and vegetables in very low amounts. An apple, for example, contains approximately 2mg of sodium.

Chloride

Chloride helps regulate fluid balance and maintain blood pressure and pH balance in the body. It's also part of stomach acid or gastric acid. The primary source of chloride is salt (sodium chloride).

There's no RDA for chloride, but the AI for males and females age 14 to 50 is 2.3g per day. The AI for males and females age 51 to 70 is 2g per day.

Toxicity hasn't been reported in humans. Chloride is excreted in urine, sweat, and feces. Food sources for chloride include table salt, sea salt, seaweed, rye, tomatoes, lettuce, and celery.

Magnesium

Magnesium is involved in maintaining bone health, and about 50 percent of the body's can be found in bone. The remaining magnesium is located in soft tissue cells where it assists with energy metabolism and a variety of other functions. Magnesium is a cofactor in hundreds of enzymes that aid in protein synthesis, glucose regulation, blood pressure regulation, and muscle and nerve functions. This mineral also participates in the active transport of calcium and potassium, which is involved in muscle contraction and blood clotting.

The RDA for magnesium for males age 19 to 30 years old is 400mg and for females 310mg. Deficiency is rare and is typically related to chronic conditions like alcoholism.

Magnesium toxicity from food sources is not possible due to the tight regulation of magnesium levels in the body by the kidneys. The tolerable UL for adults from nonfood sources is 350mg per day. However, supplementation of greater than 5,000mg per day can lead to nausea, cramping, and diarrhea.

Good sources of magnesium can be found in fibrous foods such as legumes, nuts, seeds, and whole grains. It's also found in vegetables and fruits like spinach, edamame, avocados, and bananas. Animal proteins and fish also contain magnesium.

Trace Minerals

Trace minerals include iron, iodine, chromium, molybdenum, copper, zinc, fluoride, selenium, and manganese. Your body requires these minerals in small amounts for optimal health. They're involved in many different functions, such as aiding in hormone production, bone strength, and heartbeat regulation. Your body must obtain these from your diet because it's unable to make minerals. However, it can recycle, reuse, and store some of them in your body, which is why only small amounts are required.

Iron

Iron provides many functions in your body. It's a necessary component for growth, normal cell function, and hormone and connective tissue development. It's also a key element of myoglobin and hemoglobin, which is an oxygen-carrying protein molecule found in your blood cells.

Most of the iron in your body is found in hemoglobin, with the remaining being stored in the liver, bone marrow, spleen, or muscle tissue as a part of myoglobin. Iron is stored in the form of ferritin or hemosiderin. Iron is not usually excreted through urine or feces; however, if it needs to be, it can be excreted in small amounts.

The RDA for iron for males age 19 to 50 is 8mg for males and for females 18mg. See the table at the end of this chapter for more detailed information.

Iron deficiency can be determined by a simple lab test that measures iron levels in your blood. Hemoglobin levels less than 13g/dL in men and 12g/dL in women are labeled as iron-deficiency anemia (IDA). Anemia causes symptoms of fatigue and exhaustion because without sufficient iron stores your blood can't carry enough oxygen.

Some people, like vegans who only consume plant-based foods, are at a greater risk of becoming iron deficient. This occurs because the more absorbable form of iron is called heme, which is found in animal-based foods like meat, poultry, and seafood. Plant-based foods contain nonheme iron, which is not as readily absorbed by the body. Other people at risk include pregnant women, infants and children, frequent blood donors, people with cancer, and those with GI disease or heart failure.

Iron toxicity can occur. The UL for iron for adults age 19 and older is 45mg per day.

The best sources of heme iron include lean meats such as beef, pork, chicken, and seafood. Nonheme iron can be found in nuts, vegetables, beans, and fortified grains such as cereals. Cereals or grains fortified with iron contain the most iron, with about 18mg per serving.

Zinc

Zinc is found in your body's cells. Its primary responsibility is to support your immune system, but it's also involved in cell growth and division, wound healing, taste, and smell. Zinc is a key nutrient in pregnancy and early childhood because of rapid growth and development.

The RDA for zinc for males is 11mg and for females 8mg. See the table at the end of the chapter for more detailed information.

A zinc deficiency is rare in the United States. However, it can cause stunted growth and sexual development in children and adolescents. It also causes slow wound healing, hair loss, loss of appetite, and decreased ability to taste.

The UL for zinc for adults is 40mg. Zinc taken in high amounts can be toxic and cause head-aches, nausea, vomiting, and diarrhea. It may also lead to low copper levels and decreased HDL levels.

Zinc can be found in foods that contain high amounts of protein such as beef, pork, and lamb, which all contain more zinc than fish. However, seafood such as oysters contains 73mg per serving, which is five times greater than the daily requirements. Other sources include whole grains, legumes, and nuts.

Fluoride

Fluoride is found in teeth and bones. Its primary role is mineralization of bones and teeth, which makes them stronger and protects them from decay.

There is no RDA for fluoride, but the AI for males is 3.8mg/day and for females 3.1mg/day. A deficiency of fluoride could cause dental problems such as cavities. A toxicity of fluoride is called *fluorosis*, which causes pitting and staining of teeth during tooth development and it cannot be reversed.

Fluoridated tap water is the best fluoride source in the diet. It has been shown to reduce childhood cavities by more than half. Toothpaste and mouthwash are also fortified with fluoride. Fluoride does occur naturally in some teas and seafood.

Iodine

Iodine plays a key role in thyroid function and helps produce thyroid hormones. These hormones help regulate bone formation and brain development in the fetus. They're also involved in a variety of other functions, including regulating body temperature and energy metabolism.

The RDA for iodine for adults is 150mcg. An iodine deficiency causes the thyroid gland to enlarge as it tries to collect more iodine resulting a visible protuberance in the neck called goiter. There are two types of deficiencies: a simple goiter caused from not enough iodine in the diet, and goiter caused from a deficiency or malfunction of the thyroid gland. During pregnancy, if the mother has an iodine deficiency, it will cause cretinism in the baby. Cretinism is a congenital disease that causes brain damage along with mental and physical retardation.

The UL for iodine for adults is 1,100mcg. Toxicity of iodine can also lead to goiters in adults and in a developing infant.

The best source for iodine is iodized table salt. In fact, salt is iodized to prevent goiters. Seafood such as cod, bass, perch, and haddock are high in naturally occurring iodine. Iodine can also be found in fruits and vegetables that are grown in iodine-rich soils. One fourth of a teaspoon of table salt contains 95mcg of iodine, whereas a 3-ounce serving of fish caught in the ocean contains 325mcg.

Chromium

Chromium's primary function is to enhance the action of insulin, which aids in glucose metabolism.

There's no RDA for chromium, but the AI for males age 19 to 50 is 35mcg and for females 25mcg. A deficiency of chromium will cause diabetes-like symptoms and impaired glucose utilization. There's no known toxicity for chromium.

Chromium is widely available in foods such as brewer's yeast, beef, turkey, liver, whole grains, and some fruits and vegetables. Broccoli is the best source of chromium, with 11mcg in ½ cup.

Molybdenum

Molybdenum acts as a catalyst for enzymes in the body. The RDA for molybdenum for adults is 45mcg per day. There are no known deficiencies or toxicities associated with molybdenum; however, the UL for adults is 2mg per day.

Food sources of molybdenum include legumes, nuts, whole grains, leafy greens, and liver.

Selenium

Selenium is required to protect cells from *oxidative damage.* It's also used in DNA synthesis, reproduction, and hormone metabolism. Selenium is stored in your body's muscles.

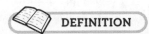 **DEFINITION**

> **Oxidative damage** (stress) is an imbalance between the body's ability to detoxify the harmful effects of free radicals and their rate of production. The body uses antioxidants to neutralize the free radicals and protect the cells.

The RDA for selenium for men is 134mg per day and for women 93mg. Selenium deficiency is rare in the United States; however, prior to the 1970s it led to Keshan disease and Keshan-Beck disease in China. Keshan disease damages the heart muscle and Keshan-Beck disease is a type of osteoarthritis that occurred in China, Tibet, and Siberia.

The UL for selenium is 400mcg per day. Toxicity called *selenosis* can occur, which can cause fatigue, skin rash, hair loss, nail loss or brittleness, garlic odor in the mouth, and a metallic taste.

The best food source of selenium is seafood. Other choices include whole grains, lean meats, poultry, and eggs. A 3-ounce portion of yellow fin tuna contains 92 mcg, which exceeds the daily requirement for this trace mineral.

Copper

Copper is found in a variety of cells and tissues in the body. Its primary function is to act as a coenzyme in all chemical reactions that involve oxygen.

The RDA for copper for adults is 900mcg per day. Copper toxicity can lead to liver damage, and the UL for adults is 10mg per day. A deficiency of copper is rare, but it can be the result of a genetic disease called *Menkes.* This disease doesn't allow the release of absorbed copper into the body. Wilson's disease is a genetic disorder that allows copper to accumulate in the liver and the brain.

Good food sources of copper are nuts, seeds, legumes, beans, whole grains, dark leafy greens, and shellfish.

Manganese

Manganese functions as a coenzyme involved in the metabolism of energy nutrients and bone formation.

There is no RDA for manganese; however, the AI for men is 2.3mg per day and for women is 1.8mg per day. Deficiency or toxicity caused by food intake is rare. Toxicity would be more likely to occur from environmental factors, such as in miners who inhale manganese dust, which leads to brain damage and nervous system disorders.

Good sources of manganese include nuts, seeds, legumes, whole grains, leafy green vegetables, and tea. A ¼ cup serving of oats contains 1.92mcg of manganese, which is 96 percent of the daily requirement for adults.

 FOODIE FACTOID

Oatmeal is known for its health benefits. It's not only a good source of fiber, but also an excellent source of manganese, molybdenum, phosphorus, and copper and a good source of magnesium, zinc, and chromium.

RDA/UL for Trace Minerals

Age/Gender	Iron	Zinc	Fluoride	Iodine	Chromium	Selenium	Copper	Manganese
Birth-6 months	.27mg	2mg	.01mg	110mcg	.2mcg	108.5 mcg	200mcg	.003mg
Infants 7-12 months	11mg	3mg	.5mg	130mcg	5.5mcg	108.5mcg	220mcg	.6mg
Children 1-3 years	7mg	3mg	.7mg	90mcg	11mcg	108.5mcg	340mcg	1.2mg
Children 4-8 years	10mg	4mg	1mg	90mcg	15mcg	108.5mcg	440mcg	1.5mg
Children 9-13 years	8mg	5mg	2mg	120mcg	21-25mcg	108.5mcg	700 mcg	1.6mg

continues

RDA/UL for Trace Minerals   (continued)

Age/Gender	Iron	Zinc	Fluoride	Iodine	Chromium	Selenium	Copper	Manganese
Males 14-18 years	11mg	11mg	3mg	150mcg	35mcg	108.5mcg	890mcg	2.2mg
Females 14 – 18 years	15mg	9mg	3mg	150mcg	24mcg	108.5mcg	890mcg	1.6mg
Males 19 and older	8mg	11mg	4mg	150mcg	35mcg	134mcg	900mcg	2.3mg
Females 19 and older	18mg	8mg	3mg	150mcg	25mcg	93mcg	900mcg	1.8mg
Pregnant women	27mg	12mg	3mg	220mcg	30mcg	60mcg	1,000mcg	2mg
Breast-feeding women	10mg	12mg	3mg	290mcg	45mcg	70mcg	1,300mcg	2.6mg

Vitamin and Mineral Supplements

The 2010 Dietary Guidelines for Americans identifies calcium, vitamin D, fiber, and potassium as nutrients that are low in everyone's diet. Ideally you should attempt to get your nutrients through food sources, but sometimes a supplement is necessary.

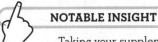 **NOTABLE INSIGHT**

Taking your supplements with food is the best way to maximize the mineral or vitamin absorption.

What Makes a Supplement Good?

The Food and Drug Administration (FDA) regulates vitamin and mineral supplements. However, manufacturers are responsible for evaluating the safety of their products. This gives companies the ability to be dishonest, so ingredients on the labels don't always match what is actually in the product. Also, manufacturers don't have to prove that the product is pure and free of contaminants. Typically, a product is only removed from the shelves after many consumer complaints and a lawsuit has been brought against the company. Here are a few key things to consider when you shop for a multivitamin supplement:

- **No more than 100 percent RDAs for vitamins and minerals:** If you're eating a variety of foods in your diet, exceeding 100 percent of the RDAs is not that beneficial and you are just paying for expensive urine.

- **USP Logo:** USP stands for the United States Pharmacopeia, which has tested this supplement and has verified that the product is pure and contains the listed ingredients in the amounts stated, will dissolve, and is made under safe and sanitary conditions.

- **Serving size:** Sometimes it may take up to four pills to meet the required amounts, which can be a problem if a person has trouble taking a large quantity of pills.

- **Additional ingredients:** Are there high amounts of herbal ingredients that are unnecessary? What are you paying for?

- **Allergens:** Are the pills free of common allergens like wheat or dairy, or are they vegetarian?

- **Type of supplement:** Is it a chewable, enteric-coated capsule or gel capsule? Some pills are coated to help them get through the acidic stomach environment without being destroyed; others like gels can be quickly absorbed. What is your goal for this supplement?

Who Needs Supplements?

Some people are at greater risk of being low in particular vitamin and minerals. This may be due to age, certain diseases, pregnancy, or avoidance of certain food groups. Supplements are recommended for the following population groups:

- Postmenopausal women: Calcium and vitamin D

- People who are on restricted diets consuming less than 1,600 calories per day

- Vegetarians who eat only plant-based foods

- People with injuries or diseases or who are on medications that interfere with nutrient absorption

- Women of childbearing age who are trying to become pregnant: folic acid

- Adults over 50: vitamin B_{12}

- Pregnant women: iron

- Breastfed infants: vitamin D

According to the CDC, more than 50 percent of all U.S. adults take multivitamin supplements. The supplement industry is a multibillion-dollar business. The National Institutes of Health (NIH) reported that the amount made from vitamin and mineral supplement sales in 2012 was approximately $13.1 billion dollars, and it increases each year.

Vitamin and mineral supplements are available for children, women, men, women and men over 50, etc. There are high-energy, high-stress, and specialty supplements to improve cardiovascular health, too. Many multivitamin supplements exceed the RDAs for nutrient values. The pills also come in micro pills, capsules, enteric-coated pills, liquid gel capsules, time-release capsules, and chewable and liquid forms. It can be a daunting process to find a supplement.

The Least You Need to Know

- Major minerals and trace minerals are found in a variety of foods and play an important role in keeping your body healthy.
- Keep iron pills away from children, as they could easily lead to a toxic overdose.
- Supplements may be used in conjunction with a healthy diet. Be sure to verify the brand you purchase contains the USP label to ensure you're getting what you paid for.
- Always check with your doctor before adding supplements to your daily regimen because some can interfere with other nutrients and medications.

Phytonutrients

The word *phytonutrient* comes from the Greek word for plant, *phyto,* and means "plant nutrients." These are additional chemical substances that offer your body a protective health benefit and help ward off disease. They're different from vitamins and minerals, but can act in a similar way.

Many phytonutrients are known to exist and scientists believe there are many more that haven't even been identified. However, research suggests there's strong evidence that phytonutrients provide a myriad of health benefits. At this time, there isn't enough research to make specific recommendations on consumption of daily amounts as with vitamin and minerals.

In this chapter, you'll learn about some of the more common phytonutrients and their potential health roles. We'll also discover which foods provide the best source for each of the phytonutrients.

In This Chapter

- The role plants play in your health
- Classification of the key phytonutrients
- The function of phytonutrients in decreasing risk of disease
- Which foods rank the highest in phytonutrients
- How your body utilizes phytonutrients

What Is a Phytonutrient?

A phytonutrient is a naturally occurring, biologically active, plant-based chemical found in all plants. It's what helps protect the plant from insects, sun damage, and disease. When we eat plants like fruit, vegetables, whole grains, herbs, and spices, we ingest those plant nutrients. Many of these active plant compounds are what give the plant its distinct color, such as carotenoids, which make carrots orange. They can also be responsible for the flavor and aroma, as with allicin in garlic and onions.

A phytonutrient is also referred to as a phytochemical, and the terms are used interchangeably. Thousands of phytonutrients exist, but only a fraction of them have been studied. Researchers have determined that some of the compounds are best consumed raw and others are more *bioavailable* when cooked, as is the case with lycopene in tomatoes.

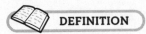 **DEFINITION**

Bioavailability refers to an active chemical compound being physiologically available for use in the body.

Phytonutrients have been used as medicine for centuries, but people didn't understand the why a certain food aided in the healing process. Scientists can now identify specific plant chemicals like lycopene and study the effects in the body or under the microscope. They also can define the compound's mode of action on specific cells in the body, such as cancerous cells.

One of the primary roles of phytonutrients is to act as antioxidants. Ongoing research is looking at the role of these plant chemicals in relation to heart disease, diabetes, cancer, and neurological diseases like Alzheimer's.

Phytonutrients are divided into three groups based on their molecular structure: phenolic acids, flavonoids, and stilbenes/lignans. Flavonoids are the largest group, and are subdivided into anthohcyanins, flavones, flavanones, isoflavones, flavonols, and flavanols. Flavonols are subdivided into catechins, epicatechins, proanthocyanidins, procyanidins, and prodelphinidins. A few of the more common phytonutrients we'll review in greater detail have been substantially researched. They are anythocyanins, lycopene, resveratrol, carotenoids, phytoestrogens, lutein, and allicin.

The Benefits of Phytonutrients

Researchers became interested in phytonutrients because they noticed a trend in epidemiological studies involving cancer and heart disease. They found that people who ate more plant-based foods tended to be healthier, have less disease, and live longer. This led them to look at the foods and their composition. Identifying one single compound and connecting it to a health claim is difficult because there may be hundreds of phytochemicals in one food. In addition, it may not be just that one phytochemical that provides the benefit, but the synergistic action of all of them combined.

One of the most beneficial roles of plant chemicals is to function as an antioxidant. Antioxidants protect your cells from damage from free radicals, which are produced during normal cell metabolism. Free radicals can also come from outside sources, such as radiation, cigarette smoke, and exposure to toxic chemicals.

According to the U.S. Department of Agriculture (USDA), phytonutrients may also support body's immune response, aid in communication between cells, kill cancer cells, repair DNA, act as a detoxifier, and alter estrogen metabolism. No recommendations for a daily intake exist because further research must be done before any conclusion can be made. Let's take a look at a few of the key phytochemicals in foods and their potential health benefits.

Carotenoids

Carotenoids contain a large subgroup of phytochemicals. Beta-carotene, lycopene, lutein, and zeaxanthin are a few that we'll discuss a little later. Researchers believe the health benefits from consuming carotenoids are due to their role as an antioxidant. Much research has been done on the role of carotenoids in relation to cancer and eye disease.

Carotenoids include more than 600 plant pigments, but they're the primary sources for orange, red, and yellow colors found in plants. Beta-carotene is also what gives the color to flamingos, goldfish, salmon, and autumn leaves. Carotenoids are fat soluble, and in order to digest them you need to have a little fat along with your carotenoid-containing food.

Beta-Carotene

Beta-carotene is a phytonutrient, but it's also the precursor to vitamin A. Your body can split beta-carotene into two molecules of vitamin A, which is an essential nutrient for your body. Beta-carotene was the first phytochemical to be measured in foods, and is found in orange, red, and yellow plant pigments.

The function of beta-carotene is to act as an antioxidant. Research has shown an ingestion of foods high in beta-carotene has aided in the prevention of vision loss due to macular degeneration, decreased the risk of breast cancer, prevented bronchitis, and decreased asthma attacks during exercise. It also has been reported to aid in pain reduction associated with osteoarthritis, decrease ovarian cancer risk, and improve muscle strength in older people.

All of this makes beta-carotene sound like a wonder nutrient. Indeed, it does have many positive effects on health, but adverse effects also have been identified through research. The most famous study is from 1994, *The Effect of Vitamin E and Beta Carotene on the Incidence of Lung Cancer and Other Cancers in Male Smokers.* In this study, the subjects were males in Finland who were supplemented with 50mg of vitamin E, 20mg of beta-carotene, or a combination of the two. The study included 29,133 male smokers age 50 to 69 years old. Researchers saw an increase in lung cancer in the subjects who were taking beta-carotene. Supplementation was stopped and the men were followed for 5 to 8 years.

After the Finland study, researchers were concerned about the negative impact of beta-carotene use on health. However, in the physician's health study, which included smokers and nonsmokers, there was no evidence that beta-carotene had an adverse affect even after 18 years of following the participants. In another study, they also reviewed the impact of beta-carotene in an antioxidant cardiovascular study of women. They found there were no beneficial effects of beta-carotene supplementation in relation to cardiovascular risk, nor did it slow age-related cognitive functions or have a negative impact.

 FOODIE FACTOID

Eating too many carrots can turn you orange. Well, actually it's yellow. This effect is typically seen in young children who can get stuck on only eating one food such as carrots. The color will eventually fade in a couple of weeks' time once the child stops eating carrots. For an adult, three large carrots per day would exceed recommended vitamin A intake and might make you turn yellow.

Food sources of beta-carotene include sweet potatoes, carrots, cantaloupe, winter squash, apricots, collard greens, kale, and broccoli. Overall, beta-carotene is a powerful antioxidant. The best bet is to consume beta-carotene–rich produce as part of a healthy diet, and you will get the added benefit of phytonutrients.

Lycopene

Lycopene belongs to the carotenoid group, and it functions as an antioxidant, too. Lycopene is a plant pigment that makes vegetables and fruit red. It has been heavily researched and studied in conjunction with the growth of cancer cells, the protective effect on bone health from free radical damage, and in relation to osteoporosis. Researchers report that eating one cup of tomatoes a day will help protect you from sun damage. That's a great motivation to include two servings of vegetables and prevent premature aging of the skin from sun exposure.

Cooking lycopene-containing foods like tomatoes has a positive effect by increasing the bio-availability of lycopene threefold. Other top food sources for lycopene are red peppers, pink grapefruit, and watermelon.

 FOODIE FACTOID

> During colonial times, tomatoes were grown only as ornamental plants. People were afraid they were poisonous because they belonged to the nightshade family of plants, *Solanaceae*. In fact, the leaves of the tomato plant are poisonous, but the fruit is not.

Lutein and Zeaxanthin

These phytonutrients are being studied in relation to vision because lutein and zeaxanthin can be stored in the retina and lens of the eye. It's believed that they can help protect your eyes from damaging ultraviolet light.

Age-related macular degeneration (AMD) is the leading cause of blindness in the elderly. Therefore, many studies examine the role of lutein in eye health. In the Age-Related Eye Disease (AREDS) study, those who took supplements of lutein and zeaxanthin had a 26 percent reduced risk of developing AMD. However, the researchers did note that those on the supplement did not consume food sources (produce) with those same phytochemicals. If it were not for the supplements, subjects would have never ingested lutein or zeaxanthin.

Additionally, the same study also looked at the effect of beta-carotene supplements opposed to lutein/zeaxanthin supplementation, and there was an 18 percent lower risk of AMD compared to the group who took beta-carotene.

Food sources of lutein and zeaxanthin include collard greens, kale, spinach, broccoli, brussels sprouts, lettuces, artichokes, and eggs. These phytonutrients are what give egg yolks, corn, and avocados their yellow color.

Flavonoids

The flavonoids are a large group of phytonutrients and are categorized as polyphenolic compounds. The common flavonoids are anthocyanidins, flavanols, flavanones, flavonols, flavones, and isoflavones. This group of phytochemicals appears to aid in cell-signaling pathways that deal with cell growth and death as opposed to working solely as an antioxidant. Research with the flavonoids has focused on their relation to cardiovascular disease, cancer, and neurodegenerative diseases.

Flavonoids vary in their chemical structure and bioavailability. Some flavonoids are attached to a sugar molecule called flavonoid glycosides. The ones not attached to a sugar molecule are flavonoid aglycones. Flavonoid glycosides are quickly broken down and absorbed in the small intestine. The remaining flavonoids may be broken down in the colon by bacterial enzymes. However, your ability to metabolize the flavonoids may depend on the overall health of your gut bacteria.

Anthocyanidins

Anthocyanidins include the dietary flavonoids cyanidin, delphinidin, malvidin, pelargonidin, peonidin, and petunidin. They're responsible for the red, blue, and purple pigments found in plants. Heat damages and breaks down these pigments, and thus decreases the biochemical activity of the anthocyanidins. It's a water-soluble molecule and is greatly affected by changes in pH. It can also be damaged by exposure to oxygen and UV light.

Research on anthocyanidins has shown they improved night vision in a study of British soldiers, prevent oxidative damage to the brain by blocking harmful chemicals from receptor sites, and prevent oxidation in LDL cholesterol in blood vessels.

Food sources of anthocyanidins include blueberries, blackberries, plums, cranberries, raspberries, red onions, red potatoes, red radishes, strawberries, beets, purple cabbage, and cherries.

Catechins

Catechins belong to the flavanol group, which is part of the larger group of flavonoids. Along with the catechins are the flavonoids epicatechin, epigalocatechin, epicatechin gallate, epigallocatechin gallate, theaflavin, and proanthocyanidins.

Chemically the catechins are very stable compounds and not adversely affected by heat or acid. They also have an astringent and bitter flavor.

Catechin is the primary phytonutrient found in tea leaves from the *Camellia sinensis* plant. Green tea is one of the most consumed beverages in the world. Observational studies have shown that consumption of three cups of tea daily may reduce the risk of heart attacks. One study in *The American Journal of Clinical Nutrition* reported that Japanese men who drank green tea containing 690mg of catechins lost more weight than the control group. Another very small study of men showed that an extract of epigallocatechin gallate (EGCG) increased the metabolic rate by 4 percent in a 24-hour period, which equated to burning an additional 65 to 200 calories.

The best food sources for catechins include quality green and white tea, cocoa, grapes, berries, and apples.

Isoflavones

Isoflavones include the flavonoids daidzein, genistein, and glycitein. Soybeans provide the most isoflavones in the diet. Only small amounts of isoflavones are found in legumes, grains, and vegetables. These phytonutrients are water-soluble, heat-stable, and are bound to sugar molecules and broken down in the small intestine. The bacterial gut flora also aids in the breakdown of the molecules.

Isoflavones have estrogen-like properties and compete for estrogen-binding sites within the cells. This makes sense because the molecular structures of isoflavones are also quite similar to human estrogen.

Research has examined the relationship between isoflavones and breast cancer, prostate cancer, menopausal symptoms, heart disease, and osteoporosis.

In 2006, the American Heart Association (AHA) reviewed 22 studies on the effect of soy protein with isoflavones finding there was only a minimal cholesterol-lowering effect or no benefit at all. Therefore, the AHA doesn't recommend isoflavone supplementation to prevent heart disease.

The primary food source for isoflavones is soy. There's approximately 200mg of isoflavones in $3^1/_2$ ounces of dried soy protein.

Resveratrol

One of the most studied stilbenes is resveratrol. Stilbenes are classified as polyphenols, which include phenolic acids, tannins, diferuloylmethanes, and flavonoids. Stilbenes have been shown to have antibacterial and antifungal properties and offer protection against heart disease.

Resveratrol is the phytochemical in red wine. The term "French Paradox" was first used by a French epidemiologist in the 1980s after researchers made the connection between the French people's high intake of cholesterol and saturated fat along with their high red wine consumption. Theoretically, the French should have a higher death rate from coronary heart disease based on their diets. However, their moderate alcohol consumption has been shown to reduce heart disease risk by 20 to 30 percent. Unfortunately, it's difficult to determine whether it was the effect of the resveratrol content or flavonoids, which are also present in red wine.

Research has also shown resveratrol to reduce platelet aggregation, decrease blood pressure, and inhibit inflammation, which is important in decreasing the risk of cardiovascular disease.

Food sources for resveratrol include the skin of grapes, red wine, purple grape juice, peanuts, and some berries.

How Phytonutrients Are Broken Down

Phytonutrients are broken down in the body according to the molecular structure of the phyto-chemical. Some phytochemicals are attached to a sugar molecule, which must be split apart. Once split, the smaller molecule can be absorbed by the small intestine. Other phytochemicals, such as beta-carotene and lycopene, require dietary fat to improve absorption because they're fat-soluble molecules, and must be emulsified by bile in the digestive process. Still others phytonutrients may require a carrier to be transported through the body. Some phytochemicals survive the pH of the stomach intact and others do not, as in the case of allicin.

Microflora in the gut are responsible for breaking down some phytochemicals. An imbalance in this bacterial colony could cause a lesser amount of certain phytochemicals (acids) to be formed. In the colon, some of the acids may be reabsorbed and travel back to the small intestine or the liver, where they're bound to another molecule before absorption into the blood.

Which Is the Best: Phytonutrient Pills or Whole Foods?

Due to all the variables in phytonutrients—from chemical structure, water-soluble/fat soluble, and damage by exposure to heat and light—it makes sense to get your phytonutrients from whole foods. Scientists are still not sure if certain phytochemicals are independent in action or if there's a synergistic effect from other plant compounds in the foods.

Another thing to consider is the extraction process of the phytonutrients into supplement form. Does the product you purchase actually contain any of the active ingredients? Has the product been tested by an independent lab to verify its contents? A supplement form may also cause an adverse reaction and be detrimental to health, as in the Finland study with beta-carotene. For example, garlic supplements have been shown to cause GI distress. Your best bet is to eat the whole foods.

Getting More Phytonutrients in Your Diet

There are no government recommendations for consuming specified amounts of phytonutrients because more research must be done in relation to health. However, eating 5 cups of fruits and vegetables daily and making sure half your plate is filled with colorful fruits and vegetables is a good start.

Phytonutrients in Foods

As we learned with some phytonutrients like lycopene, it's important to eat a variety of cooked and raw foods. The following table provides top food sources and amounts for select phytochemicals.

Phytonutrient	Serving	Food Sources	Amount per Serving mg
Beta-carotene	1 cup	Carrot juice, canned	22.0
	1 cup	Pumpkin, canned	17.0
	1 cup	Spinach, frozen, cooked	13.8
	1 medium	Sweet potato, baked	13.1
	1 cup	Kale, frozen, cooked	11.5
Lycopene	1 cup	Tomato purée, canned	54.4
	1 cup	Tomato juice, canned	2.0
	Slice ($^1/_{16}$ of whole)	Watermelon, raw	13.0
	1 cup	Tomatoes, raw	4.6
	$^1/_2$ each	Pink grapefruit	1.7
Lutein/Zeaxanthin	1 cup	Spinach, frozen, cooked	29.8
	1 cup	Kale, frozen, cooked	25.6
	1 cup	Collards, frozen, cooked	18.5
	1 cup	Summer squash, cooked	4.9
	1 cup	Peas, frozen, cooked	3.8
Anthocyanin	3.5 ounces	Blackberries	89-211
	3.5 ounces	Blueberries	67-183
	3.5 ounces	Red grapes	25-92
	3.5 ounces	Strawberries	15-75
	5 ounces	Red wine	1-35

From the Linus Pauling Institute.

Colorful Eating

When it comes to phytonutrients, your goal is to eat more fruits, vegetables, and whole grains, and consider adding green tea and cocoa to your diet. Be sure half of your plate is made up of colorful fruits and vegetables.

Phytonutrients Recipe

The following recipe is a good source of phytonutrients.

Beet Salsa

Yield:	Prep Time:	Cook time:	Serving Size:
2 cups	20 minutes	35 minutes	$1/2$ cup
Each serving has:			
60 calories	4g total fat	0g saturated fat	0mg cholesterol
270mg sodium	6g carbohydrate	2g fiber	0g protein

1 lb. red beets	$1/2$ red onion, finely chopped
1 TB. vegetable oil	1 TB. lime juice
$1/4$ tsp. kosher salt	Zest of 1 lime
1 large jalapeno, seeded and finely chopped	$1/4$ tsp. kosher salt
	2 TB. cilantro, finely chopped

1. Preheat oven to 400°F. Remove roots and tops from each beet.

2. Peel beets and cut into $1/4$-inch pieces. Toss beets in oil and salt. Place on baking sheet and roast for 20-25 minutes or until tender. Remove from oven and let cool.

3. Combine cooled beets, jalapeno, red onion, lime juice, lime zest, salt, and cilantro. Mix well. Refrigerate until serving or serve immediately at room temperature.

Cook's note: Wear disposable gloves when working with red beets to prevent staining. For a spicier dish, use some of the seeds from the jalapeno.

The Least You Need to Know

- Phytonutrients are attributed to disease protection in diets high in fruits and vegetables.

- Scientific evidence does not support claims that phytochemical supplements are as beneficial as whole foods.

- Research is ongoing when it comes to phytonutrients, and much more time and research is needed before scientists can identify all their effects on your health.

- Eating a variety of cooked and raw colorful produce is the best natural way to achieve a high level of phytonutrients in your diet.

Making Your Best Food Choices

Before you can make a change toward good nutrition, you need to know what the best foods are for you to choose from. In this part, we walk you through all the major food groups: fruits, vegetables, whole grains, proteins, dairy, and fats. You'll learn what nutrients each group provides and their vital role in your body.

We'll also learn how to read food labels and understand packaging claims. We'll explain what a supply chain is, in addition to the differences between additives and genetically modified foods (GMOs). We also take a look at the journey of food from the farm to the table and explain the differences between organic and conventionally grown produce. Finally, we will help you make the best possible choice for you and your family when it comes to cooking oils and their impacts on health.

CHAPTER 12

Understanding Your Foods

Identifying what foods to choose and in the right amounts to create a healthy diet for yourself can be a daunting task. But with a little practice you'll come to learn how easy eating healthier can be. When it comes to good health, eating a variety of foods every day helps ensure your body will have access to all the nutrients it needs.

In this chapter, we'll review the vital nutrients in each of the food groups and why you need them to support a healthy body. We'll also look at where to find additional nutrients and learn how to read the food label.

In This Chapter

* Eating for health from all the food groups
* The best way to replace lost nutrients from certain food groups
* Consumer regulations surrounding food labels
* How to get the most information from food labels

What Should I Eat?

The contents of your grocery cart should reflect your plate. The Dietary Guidelines for Americans call for consuming fruits, vegetables, whole grains, low-fat and fat-free dairy, and lean meats and seafood. Fill your plate with at least 50 percent fruits and vegetables and divide the remaining portion between lean proteins and whole grains with dairy on the side to satisfy these recommendations. Keep these guidelines in mind when you fill your cart to ensure you take home the types of foods you should be eating on a daily basis.

The Basic Food Groups

Food is divided into five basic food groups based on their similarities in nutrient content. Fruits, vegetables, whole grains, lean proteins, and dairy make up the diverse nutrient groups. Eating a variety of foods within each food group ensures you consume all the nutrients your body needs to function and to ward off disease.

Whole Grains

Whole grains are ones that have been minimally processed, leaving the grain and its nutrient profile intact. According to the Whole Grain Council, in order to be considered a whole grain, all parts of the grain must be present. The parts consist of 100 percent of the bran, germ, and endosperm in the whole kernel.

Recommendations include eating *at least* half of your grains from whole grain sources. Eventually, choosing mostly whole grains rather then refined grains is a health-minded goal. Refined grains are often enriched with the vitamins they lose during processing. The information you'll find on the nutrition label may read similar to the unrefined varieties. However, the nutrition you may receive from the added nutrients can actually be less than those that would actually come from whole grains. Many refined grains also contain added fat and sugar. Some grains may appear to be whole but have been processed. Watch for the word *pearled* on products such as farro and barley; it indicates the grain has been processed.

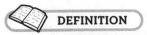 **DEFINITION**

A grain that has been **pearled** has had the outer portion polished. This process removes the bran and results in a grain no longer considered whole even though it still contains the endosperm and germ.

Ample scientific evidence exists to support the correlation between increased whole grain intake and reduction in some forms of cancer, obesity, cardiovascular disease, and type 2 diabetes. Whole grains are rich in vitamins, minerals, and antioxidants, including B vitamins, iron, magnesium, phosphorus, and fiber.

Whole grains help you feel full longer and slow the release of insulin. Fiber from whole grains adds bulk and absorbs water, aiding in the digestion process. Vitamins in whole grains aid in energy production and the metabolism of the food you eat.

Whole grains contain amino acids in varying degrees. Some grains are considered complete proteins because they include all nine essential amino acids in adequate proportions. Some whole grains lack sufficient quantities of a few amino acids, making them incomplete. The amino acid lysine is generally lacking or in a lower proportion to the other amino acids in whole grains. By including items in your diet high in lysine (beans, legumes, and soy), you'll make the whole grain a complete protein.

Grains that are considered complete proteins include quinoa, amaranth, millet, and buckwheat.

If you're following a gluten-free diet, there's no need to avoid all grains. Only grains from wheat, barley, and rye should be completely excluded. Some grains (especially oats) may be processed in plants with wheat and may contain trace levels. Check the packaging to ensure they're considered gluten-free.

The following grains are considered gluten-free:

- Amaranth
- Buckwheat
- Corn
- Millet
- Quinoa

- Brown rice
- Sorghum
- Teff
- Wild rice
- Oats

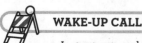 **WAKE-UP CALL**

Instant oatmeal has been cut into smaller pieces and has disodium phosphate added to decrease cooking time. The addition of disodium phosphate makes this product undesirable for those watching their sodium intake. Many types of instant oatmeal also have added sugar. Instant oatmeal is still considered a whole grain, but it has a higher glycemic index than other oatmeal products due to the small particle size. Quick-cooking, old-fashioned, and steel-cut oats are all nutritionally equivalent.

Make smart choices when selecting products such as breads and cereals, as misleading labeling runs rampant in the grains aisle. You'll find that many product labels claim "Whole Grain," "Ancient Grain," "Grain and Seed," or "7 Grain." However, you must read the item's ingredients list to know for sure if the product is 100 percent whole grain or whole wheat. If the first ingredient is whole-wheat flour, the bread is truly made with whole wheat. If the first ingredient is enriched wheat flour, it's not considered whole grain, but rather is made primarily or solely from processed flour. If the product claims it's rich in whole grain or whole wheat, the terms "refined" or "processed" must not come before the word "whole." Apply this principle to all cereal and bread products as well.

Making the transition from refined grains to whole can take some time. If you've always eaten white rice and pasta, slowly start converting to brown rice and pasta by mixing white and whole grain together. Finding new recipes that incorporate whole grains is helpful as well.

Adding whole grains into your dietary pattern can be simple. A serving is considered 1 ounce. This equals to about a half cup of cooked whole grains, one small slice of bread, or one cup of ready-to-eat cereal. Keep in mind that whole grains take longer to cook than refined grains. Planning ahead will make adding them to your diet easier.

If you find yourself short on time, cook whole grains ahead of time and freeze them in serving sizes for last-minute dinners. Look for precooked bags of quinoa, brown and wild rice, and mixed grains. These are easy to microwave and are shelf stable until opened. Try new varieties of grains such as bulgur, farro, quinoa, and barley as substitutes for rice and pasta. Whole grains are great incorporated into salads or on top of Greek yogurt and cottage cheese.

Protein

Protein is an integral component of muscles. Further, protein acts in every cellular function in your body. Animal protein is generally high in B vitamins, vitamin E, iron, zinc, and magnesium. Plant-based proteins are a good source of thiamin, riboflavin, niacin, phosphorous, potassium, and fiber. Some protein sources such as fish, nuts, and seeds are excellent sources of the essential fatty acids omega-3 and omega-6. Consuming adequate protein during an illness or the aging process ensures maintaining lean body mass, especially since it's metabolically active.

Protein in your diet may come from both animal and plant sources. As previously mentioned, whole grains provide protein, whether it be complete as in peanuts, or incomplete. The most biologically available sources of protein are animal proteins such as meat, seafood, eggs, and dairy.

The biological value (BV) of protein is based on the amount of nitrogen absorbed from the protein. Eggs have 100 percent BV. Most animal protein sources are about 97 percent digestible, and plant-based proteins are between 70 and 90 percent digestible.

Many Americans eat more protein than is needed to maintain both muscle and vascular protein stores. Keep serving sizes in check to ensure that extra protein isn't consumed and converted into fat. An amount equal in size to a deck of cards is considered a 3- to 4-ounce serving of meat and would contain approximately 7 grams of protein per ounce (21-28 grams).

With a high BV, eggs are perfect for any meal. Eggs can be poached and placed on toast, tossed over a salad, or scrambled and served alongside roasted vegetables. Keep hard-boiled eggs on hand for a midafternoon snack. Eggs are versatile and quick cooking, and can even be cooked and reheated in a microwave. Do a little online research and practice your cooking technique.

Fruits and Vegetables

Filling half your plate with fruits and vegetables will ensure you consume adequate amounts of the vitamins and minerals needed to maintain a healthy body. The U.S. Department of Agriculture (USDA) reports the most under-consumed nutrients are vitamins A, C, and K; folate; magnesium; potassium; and fiber. Fruits and vegetables are high in these nutrients.

Eating a diet rich in fruits and vegetables has been scientifically proven to reduce the risk of cardiovascular disease, some cancers, obesity, and type 2 diabetes. Filling up on these nutrient-packed foods will help you eat proper portions of the other food groups and aid in a balanced diet.

Fruits and vegetables are also packed with phytonutrients. Different colors are higher in different antioxidants and nutrients. Be sure to select a wide variety of colors when choosing what fruits and veggies to eat. The array of colors will ensure you get all the nutrients you need to keep as healthy as possible.

Fresh fruits and vegetables can be a large portion of your food budget. With some guidelines, you can always have some on hand. Always shop for produce that's in season, which is usually advertised and less expensive. Plan to use items that spoil quicker at the beginning of the week like berries and leafy greens. Produce such as apples, bananas, oranges, carrots, and potatoes have a longer shelf life. Finally, with portable and preprepped fruits and vegetables available in the produce section, there's no reason not to include them in your meals.

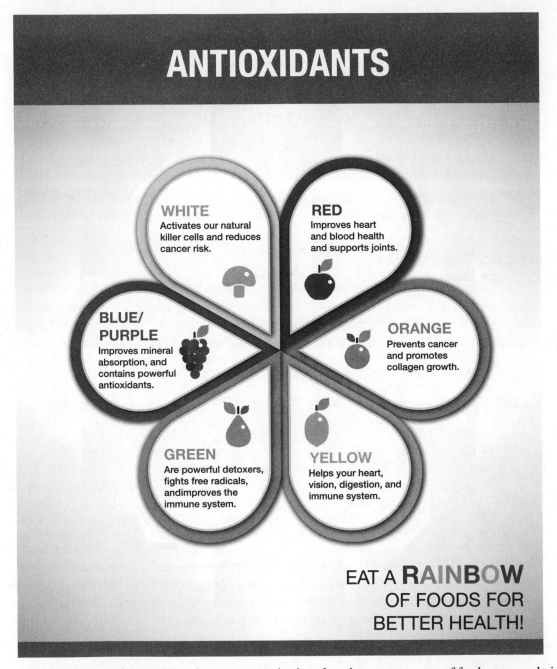

ANTIOXIDANTS

WHITE
Activates our natural killer cells and reduces cancer risk.

RED
Improves heart and blood health and supports joints.

BLUE/PURPLE
Improves mineral absorption, and contains powerful antioxidants.

ORANGE
Prevents cancer and promotes collagen growth.

GREEN
Are powerful detoxers, fights free radicals, andimproves the immune system.

YELLOW
Helps your heart, vision, digestion, and immune system.

EAT A **RAINBOW** OF FOODS FOR BETTER HEALTH!

Canned fruits and vegetables also are a great backup for when you run out of fresh ones or their price are high. Look for varieties with reduced sodium and rinse them well before heating. When you select canned fruits, be sure they are packed in their own juice without any added sugar. Once the cans are open, be sure to store the contents in a refrigerator-safe container. Leaving them in the can may alter the taste.

Frozen fruits and vegetables picked at their peak of freshness are a wonderful solution. Items can be kept in your freezer for months and pulled out when you've eaten up your fresh purchases. Frozen fruits and vegetables are also great in smoothies and stir-fries.

 WAKE-UP CALL

> Food cans and plastic bottles are lined with an epoxy containing the chemical BHA. The FDA believes BHA is safe, but they're continuously researching to determine if it's leaching into the contents. They're also looking at what health detriments it may be causing. If you're concerned about the possible effects of BHA, look for containers that are labeled BHA-free. Keeping bottles and cans out of the heat will also reduce the likelihood of BHA contaminating the food.

Dairy

Dairy products are an excellent source of calcium, vitamin D, and potassium. Some dairy products, such as kefir and Greek yogurt, contain probiotics. Generally, low-fat and nonfat milk and yogurt are recommended due to the lower saturated fat content. If you're choosing nondairy alternatives such as almond or soy, be sure you choose unsweetened varieties that are fortified with calcium and vitamin D. Dairy milk is a great source of protein, but not all alternatives contain protein. Be sure to read the nutrition facts label.

Cheese, like other dairy products, is a good source of protein. Use cheese in moderation and opt for strong-flavored cheeses like feta, blue, or Parmesan to add to salads. If you're a cheese lover, splurge on a different kind from the gourmet cheese section in your store once a month. The flavors are unsurpassable, and you can eat a slice or two a day as a snack along with apples, grapes, or a handful of nuts.

Processed cheese is a blend of cheeses with the addition of disodium phosphate. Often processed cheese will not contain enough true cheese to be labeled as cheese and may be referred to as a cheese food. They also have additional added oils and may be much higher in calories.

Greek yogurt and cottage cheese are also a great source of protein and supply needed calcium. Look for low-fat or nonfat options without added sugar. Cottage cheese can be high in sodium, so be sure to compare the brands when making your selections. Add fruits, nuts, and ground flaxseed to your yogurt. Use cottage cheese to add protein to your salads or to top a baked potato. Nonfat plain Greek yogurt is a great alternative to sour cream and provides more protein and less fat.

Healthy Fats

Healthy fats can help brain function, slow down cognitive decline, and help maintain optimal cholesterol levels. Choose fat sources that are liquid at room temperature. Use monounsaturated fats such as olive oil in place of butter. Eat unsalted nuts and seeds high in omega-3s.

Fish is an excellent source of omega-3 fatty acids. Eat fatty fish such as salmon, mackerel, tuna, sardines, anchovies, and rainbow trout in 4-ounce portion sizes, two to four times a week. The University of Michigan Integrative Health department recommends a ratio of two to four times as much omega-3 in your diet as omega-6.

What If I Eliminate Food Groups?

Oftentimes, eliminating foods may be necessary due to allergies or religious or social beliefs. Eliminating specific foods will not generally cause problems in maintaining a balanced diet. However, when entire food groups are eliminated, the nutrients readily available in that group must be added to the diet in other ways. Being aware of your reasons for eliminating entire groups and making efforts to replace those lost ingredients will help alleviate any nutritional deficiencies.

Dairy Alternatives

Many individuals who are lactose intolerant can't tolerate any dairy foods. For them, consumption of lactose causes cramping, gas, and diarrhea due to their body producing very small amounts of the enzyme lactase needed to break down lactose. Lactose-intolerant people, however, may be able to consume yogurt in small amounts due to the yogurt's probiotics, which have already broken down some of the lactose. Additionally, the probiotics will aid in supporting a healthy gut environment, which will help with digestion. Hard and aged cheeses, such as Swiss and cheddar, have low lactose levels and may also be tolerated. If you've eliminated dairy altogether due to lactose intolerance, try slowly adding hard cheeses, yogurt, and dairy back into your diet a bite at a time to help build up a tolerance.

> **NOTABLE INSIGHT**
>
> Lactose intolerance is a condition that often affects individuals as they age. The National Library of Medicine estimates 30 million Americans will have some degree of lactose intolerance by the age of 20. Trauma to the GI tract may cause transitory lactose intolerance, which often subsides as the gut returns to normal functioning. In rare instances, babies may be born with a genetic defect that makes it impossible for their body to produce the lactase enzyme.

Products that contain the lactase enzyme may also be an option for those with lactose intolerance. These lactase-added enzymes also break down the lactose disaccharide into two monosaccharides for ease of digestion. Lactaid milk has a similar nutrition profile to fat-free milk. Yogurt, cottage cheese, and other dairy products are available in Lactaid versions.

Milk alternatives are plentiful if you choose to not drink dairy milk. Soy, almond, coconut, and rice milk are all readily available. Since these options aren't animal-based, their nutrient profile will differ. Many alternatives fortify their products with calcium, protein, and vitamin D to make them more comparable to dairy milk. Be sure the option you choose doesn't have added sugar.

Gluten-Free Alternatives

Individuals with celiac disease must avoid foods containing gluten due to the inability to digest gliadin, a protein found in gluten. Other individuals have medically diagnosed gluten sensitivity without having the antibody for celiac disease. These individuals may experience symptoms similar to celiac disease without the intestinal damage. Other individuals follow a gluten-free diet due to the "health halo" gluten-free products currently have.

Oftentimes individuals "feel better" when they stop consuming gluten, because they're giving up refined carbohydrates along with the added sugar and fat that accompanies so many products containing gluten. Keep in mind that gluten grains generally are not the culprit for those without medically diagnosed sensitivity or allergies. Switching to only whole-grain products without added sugar and fat may have the same benefits.

Due to trends and consumer demand for gluten-free products, following a gluten–free diet is not as obtrusive as it once was. For example, pastas made with quinoa or brown rice are readily available. The wide availability of less-common grains like quinoa and amaranth has also given those avoiding gluten-containing grains more options.

There are gluten free flour alternatives for the home baker. The flours use a combination of rice flour, cornstarch, milk powder, tapioca flour, potato starch, and *xanthan gum*.

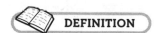 **DEFINITION**

> **Xanthan gum** is an ingredient often used in gluten-free foods. It's a polysaccharide made by bacteria. Xanthan gum is used as a food additive and acts as a stabilizer and thickener. In 1963, it was approved for food use after undergoing extensive safety testing. It's on the FDA's list of approved food additives.

Reading food packages has become simpler due to the FDA's definition of gluten-free. According to the FDA, if products are labeled gluten-free, they must either inherently be gluten-free or not contain or be made from a gluten grain. All products labeled as gluten-free must contain less than 20 parts per million of gluten. This labeling is voluntary and food producers aren't required to label their foods as gluten-free.

Food Combining

Foods are generally eaten in combination with other foods at one sitting or at some point in the same day. Some food groups need a complementary food in order for it to be considered "whole." As discussed in Chapter 7, most plant-based proteins are not complete proteins and lack sufficient amounts of the amino acid lysine. To make them a complete protein, you should eat a second protein high in the amino acids they lack. For example, beans are low in the amino acid methionine and rice is low in lysine. If eaten together or in the same day, the shortcomings of one food make up for the other.

Traditionally, two complementary foods are often served together. Beans and rice, hummus and a pita, and a peanut butter sandwich are all examples of successful pairings to make up what is known as complete proteins.

The Food Label

The Food and Drug Administration (FDA) is responsible for ensuring foods sold in the United States are safe for consumption. The two main laws that outline how foods should be labeled are the Food, Drug, and Cosmetic Act (FD&C Act) and the Fair Packaging and Labeling Act (FP&L Act). The Nutrition Labeling and Education Act (NLEA) then amended the FD&C Act. These regulations lay out standards and claims allowed on labels. All labeling must be done with the intention to not deceive the customer.

The nutrition facts label, as we know it today, was mandated in 1993. Only small changes have been made over the past two decades, and it's in need of reform to reflect how consumers today use the information provided. Proposed changes include new actual serving sizes, added sugar, amounts of vitamin D and potassium, and removing "calories from fat" information due to the lack of usefulness. The label will also get a new look with calories highlighted, shifting %DV to the left, and additional reconfiguration for consumer ease.

Nutrition Facts
Serving Size 1 cup (228g)
Servings Per Container about 2

Amount Per Serving

Calories 250	Calories from Fat 110

	% Daily Value*
Total Fat 12g	18%
Saturated Fat 3g	15%
Trans Fat 3g	
Cholesterol 30mg	10%
Sodium 470mg	20%
Total Carbohydrate 31g	10%
Dietary Fiber 0g	0%
Sugars 5g	
Proteins 5g	

Vitamin A	4%
Vitamin C	2%
Calcium	20%
Iron	4%

* Percent Daily Values are based on a 2,000 calorie diet. Your Daily Values may be higher or lower depending on your calorie needs:

	Calories:	2,000	2,500
Total Fat	Less than	65g	80g
Saturated Fat	Less than	20g	25g
Cholesterol	Less than	300mg	300mg
Sodium	Less than	2,400mg	2,400mg
Total Carbohydrate		300g	375g
Dietary Fiber		25g	30g

For educational purposes only. This label does not meet the labeling requirements described in 21 CFR 101.9.

The nutrition facts panel or food label is designed to help you understand how a food fits into your diet by providing information on serving size, calories, fats, and key vitamins and minerals.
Courtesy of the U.S. Food and Drug Administration.

Labeling

The NLEA was added to the regulations to require that food be labeled with basic nutrition information and health messages. Packaging must also include the name and address of the distributor, producer, or manufacturer.

According to the FDA, the label must include what the product is (name) and how much of the product is in the package (amount). Size and font type as well as location of required information is specified according to the package type. Not all information will be in the exact same location on every food package.

Each food product must contain a list of ingredients. Ingredients should be listed in order by weight, meaning the ingredient in the largest proportion in the product is the first listed. The ingredients in the smallest proportion are listed last. Ingredients are noted by their common name known by consumer, not the scientific name. If an approved chemical ingredient is used in the product, the common name and use should both be listed (e.g., "ascorbic acid to promote color retention"). Allergen terms must also be included.

 NOTABLE INSIGHT

The following must *always* be labeled on foods:

- Alcohol
- Aspartame for those with phenylketonuria (PKU)
- Sulfites
- Monosodium glutamate (MSG)

One of the not-so-healthy things you need to be cognizant of is that trans fat listed as 0 grams may actually contain up to 0.5 grams by law due to rounding regulations. Read the ingredients list and if hydrogenated oil or partially hydrogenated oil is listed, then the product contains some trans fats.

The Serving Size

The serving size listed on the nutrition facts label is often very different from what you may consider an actual serving. Don't assume an entire package or container of an item is one serving. The serving size is noted at the top of the nutrition facts label. The size should be listed in units the consumer can relate to, such as cup or tablespoon. The common measurement is followed by a metric measurement. In addition to serving size, you should note how many servings are included in the package. This may give you a better idea of how much of the product you can eat at one sitting.

New guidelines have been proposed for changes in serving sizes. In the last two decades since the creation of the nutrition facts label, serving sizes have grown. The FDA recognizes this and is moving toward mandating that serving sizes be more reflective of the quantity consumed at one sitting. A small bag of chips may currently be four servings. With the new proposed regulation, the entire bag would become one serving. Nutrition facts labels may indicate what the nutrition facts are for the entire bag along with a smaller portion, such as 1 cup.

What Is % Daily Value?

Based on a 2,000-calorie diet, the % daily value (%DV) is the recommendation for key nutrients. Using the percentages along the right-hand side of the nutrition facts label, you can determine if the product is a good source of the key nutrients. For items you would want to limit, such as saturated fat, cholesterol, and sodium, having a %DV of 5% or less is ideal. For those you would want more of, such as fiber, vitamins, and minerals, 20% or more is ideal. "Good Source" foods must provide 10 to 19% of the daily value of whatever they are a good source.

You can use the %DV to compare similar products for a quick reference as to which product is higher in calcium or fiber. Be sure you're comparing equal serving sizes. Instead of looking for words that may be misleading such as "light" or "low-fat," read the %DV and see for yourself.

Not all nutrients have a %DV. Protein-containing products must contain one if the product makes a label claim about the amount of protein such as being "high-protein." No daily value has been set as acceptable intake for sugar. The amount of sugar included on the nutrition facts label includes sugars occurring naturally as well as added sugar. However, there is a push for labels to differentiate between the two types of sugar.

Packaging Claims

There are three types of claims allowed by the government that manufacturers can make on their labels: nutrient claims, health claims, and structure/function claims. Each type has specific requirements associated with its use. Let's take a look at each type of the legal claims that can be made on products.

Nutrient Claims

Nutrient claims relate to actual nutrient or implied levels. Examples of claims include "low fat," "reduced calorie," or "100 calories." Claims are usually only for nutrients that have daily value % daily value associated with them. The FDA has specific nutrient claims allowed on packaging. Any claim not on the list is not allowed.

Relative nutrient claims compare the amount in the product to a reference food. These statements include terms such as "light," "reduced," "added," "more," or "less." Other nutrient claims such as "high," "lean," and "antioxidant" have specific definitions tied to them.

If a nutrient claim is made on a product, generally a disclosure must be included if the product contains more than 13 grams total fat, 4 grams saturated fat, 60 milligrams cholesterol, or 480 milligrams sodium, for example. These nutrient levels are considered above the Reference Amount Customarily Consumed (RACC). Allowed nutrient levels for meals are higher. The disclosure statement helps eliminate any possibility the claim will be misleading to the consumer.

Health claims may be printed on food packages, are strictly regulated, and must be approved by the FDA before use. A health claim is when the benefit of a product is linked to a disease or condition. The claim may be explicitly stated ("Diets low in saturated fat and cholesterol that include 25 grams of soy protein a day may reduce the risk of heart disease") or be implied (such as the heart symbol). Claims may only apply to prevention, not treatment or cure of diseases.

The following table provides a description of what the words found on a label mean.

Nutrient	Free	Low	Reduced/Less	Other
Calories	Less than 5 calories per serving	40 calories or less per serving. Meals less than 120 calories per serving	At least 25% fewer calories per serving than reference food	"Light" or "Lite." If 50% or more calories from fat, then fat must be reduced by 50%.
Total fat	Less than 0.5g fat per serving	Less than 3g fat per serving	At least 25% less fat per serving than reference food	
Saturated fat & trans fat	Less than 0.5g saturated or trans fat per serving	Less than 1g saturated fat per serving or less than 15% of calories from saturated fat	At least 25% less saturated fat per serving than reference food	
Cholesterol	Less than 2mg cholesterol per serving	Less than 20mg cholesterol per serving	At least 25% less cholesterol per serving than reference food	No claims about cholesterol allowed if product has greater than 2g saturated fat

continues

continued

Nutrient	Free	Low	Reduced/Less	Other
Sodium	Less than 5mg sodium per serving	Less than 140mg sodium per serving	At least 25% (50% for "light") less sodium per serving than reference food	"Very low sodium" must be less than 35mg of sodium per serving.
Salt	No salt added during processing	"Lightly salted" means 50% less sodium added than reference food.		
Sugar	Less than .5g sugar per serving	No definition	At least 25% less sugar per serving than reference food	"No sugar added" means no sugar-containing ingredients were added.

Adapted from *FDA Guidance for Industry: Food Labeling Guide*.

Health Claims

Another category of claims food companies can make about their products are health claims. The FDA strictly regulates these particular types of claims. Health claims are made when a food or ingredient of the food has a relationship with a disease or health condition. These claims have science backing them up and have also been reviewed by the FDA. Health claims have two parts to them. The first is the food or food substance, and the second is the disease or health condition.

 NOTABLE INSIGHT

Oftentimes food companies will petition the FDA for new health claims. The FDA will review the scientific evidence to determine if enough evidence is available to draw health conclusions. If the FDA finds enough evidence to support the health claim, it's approved and will subsequently be added to the list. If the evidence is weak or lacking, the FDA will deny the petition.

The following is a list of the approved health claims. Only these links between food or food substances and listed disease or health condition may be made.

- Calcium and a reduced risk of osteoporosis
- Calcium and vitamin D and a reduced risk of osteoporosis

- Dietary fat and a reduced risk of cancer

- Diets low in sodium and a reduced risk of hypertension

- Diets low in saturated fat and cholesterol and a reduced risk of coronary heart disease

- Fiber-containing grain products, grains, fruits, and vegetables and a reduced risk of cancer

- Fruits, vegetables, and grain products that contain fiber, particularly soluble fiber, and a reduced risk of coronary heart disease

- Fruits and vegetables and a reduced risk of cancer

- Folate and a reduced risk of neural tube defects

- Dietary noncarcinogenic carbohydrates and sweeteners does not promote dental caries

- Soluble fiber from certain foods and a reduced risk of coronary heart disease

- Soy protein and a reduced risk of coronary heart disease

- Plant sterol/sterol esters and a reduced risk of coronary heart disease

- Whole grain foods and a reduced risk of heart disease and certain cancers

- Whole gain foods with moderate fat content and a reduced risk of heart disease

- Potassium and a reduced risk of high blood pressure and stroke

- Fluorinated water and a reduced risk of dental caries

- Diets low in saturated fat, cholesterol, and trans fat may reduce the risk of heart disease

- Substitution of saturated fat in the diet with unsaturated fatty acids may reduce the risk of heart disease

Structure and Function Claims

The structure and function claims category made on food labels describes how a nutrient or food will affect the healthy structure or ability of the body to function. These claims don't need to be approved by the FDA and are not preapproved. However, the product must also state the food will not "diagnose, treat, cure, or prevent any disease." According to the FDA, structure/function claims are phrases such as "calcium builds strong bones" or "fiber maintains bowel regularity."

The Least You Need to Know

- Eating a balanced diet consists of eating proper portions and combinations of foods from all of the five basic food groups.

- If you eliminate entire food groups, do your homework to determine how you can make up for missing nutrients.

- Food labels are intended to give you the information necessary to make smart and healthy choices.

- Learning how to read the nutrition facts label will help you compare foods, moderate your portions, and estimate your daily intake.

Best Shopping Practices

With every purchase you make at the grocery store, you're supporting an industry. Industry practices vary greatly between each farmer or rancher and whether or not they're classified as an organic or a conventional facility. These businesses that bring food to the marketplace can impact the environment and the safety of your food.

In this chapter, we'll learn the difference between what the words "organic" and "conventionally grown" really mean. We will also review the supply chain process and find out how food is kept safe on its way to you. Additionally we will look into the use of genetically modified organisms and food additives.

In This Chapter

- From the farm to the marketplace
- Defining organic foods and products
- Examining the role of additives in food
- Unraveling genetically modified organisms
- What's all the buzz about sustainable farming?
- How to select safe and healthy foods

Safe Food Choices

One in six Americans will experience a foodborne illness each year, according to the Centers for Disease Control and Prevention (CDC). Over 3,000 Americans will die as a result. According to a report from the U.S. Department of Agriculture (USDA) in 2014, the estimated cost of foodborne illnesses is over $15.6 billion. Keeping the food supply and food served safe is critical to public health.

Supply Chain

Food can travel great distances to reach the consumer in the marketplace. Food starts on its journey with the farmer or rancher. Many farmers and ranchers use *co-operatives (co-ops)* that purchase their products and handle them in larger volume. Co-ops generally sell the products to processors. If farmers and ranchers don't use co-ops, the products will likely go directly to processors. During each step of the process, risk of contamination is always present.

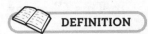 **DEFINITION**

> **Cooperatives (co-ops)** are owned and operated by a group of members with a common interest and for the benefit of all members and their community. According to the National Council of Farmer Cooperatives, farmers get a percentage of the net profits reflecting their contribution of products to the co-op. Co-ops have been working with farmers and have been part of the rural farmer's foundation for over 100 years.

Processors or manufacturers are the next link in the supply chain. They take raw goods and alter them to add value and convenience for the consumer. This is generally where food is packaged and labeled.

After processing, foods then move on to the distributor. It's the distributor's job to deliver the finished products in a safe and timely manner to suppliers for retail buyers. Distributors may carry a wide range of products or a very narrow selection, such as only dairy, produce, or meat. Some distributors skip the suppliers altogether and deliver directly to the customer, restaurant, or store.

Once the products are received by the supplier from the distributor, the supplier fills orders placed by customers. Suppliers may specialize in food service or grocery items. Facilities such as restaurants, grocery stores, and other food-related retail outlets order and receive products from the supplier with set delivery dates and times.

According to the Harvard School of Public Health, each part of the food supply chain is dependent on the other parts. When one part experiences problems, the others follow suit. Such problems in the food supply chain generally result in higher prices to consumers.

Keeping Food Safe

In this constantly growing world, our food supply must change to keep up with technology. Ensuring a safe supply is vital to our health. Research is continually evolving to find new ways and technology to secure the supply. According to IBM Research, securing a safe food supply starts as early as soil testing, and the food is rigorously tested along the way until it reaches the consumer.

Maintaining an efficient and time-based supply chain is imperative for food safety. Reputable distributors and retailers ensure food received from manufacturers or producers is kept and transported in a safe manner. If distributors don't follow proper temperature and time controls, it's at their expense. Many shipping and receiving facilities at manufacturers, distributors, and retailers check temperatures on items as they're received and shipped out. Facility workers are trained to take notice of packaging damage or deterioration and signs of temperature abuse. Such items are then refused. Highly sensitive products, such as seafood, often have temperature strips attached to packaging inside trucks showing the lowest and highest temperature the package experienced during transport.

Current local health codes require routine inspections to ensure that facilities where food is prepared and stored are clean. Sanitation standards are designed to reduce the risk associated with the preparation and storage of food.

Organic vs. Conventionally Grown

Organic products are those created with concern for the environment and without using products that don't occur naturally, such as antibiotics and pesticides. Conventionally grown crops use pesticides, synthetic chemical fertilizers, herbicides, and genetically modified organisms (GMOs). Conventional farming, in turn, allows for greater crop yields with less manual labor and hence a lower price.

Organic farmers and ranchers strive to leave the smallest *carbon footprint* possible while preserving animal welfare. Organic products benefit the farmers and ranchers who able to offer these products at higher prices. According to the USDA, consumers spend over $35 million dollars annually on organic products.

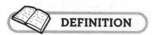

DEFINITION

A common term in the sustainability world is **carbon footprint.** This refers to the amount of pressure on the environment caused by the creation of or use of particular product or system. The footprint is measured by the amount of greenhouse gasses emitted in relation to said product or system. There are several online calculators consumers can use to estimate their carbon footprint.

The USDA has developed three levels of organic labeling:

- **100% organic:** Must not contain any portion of any product that's not 100 percent organic.

- **Organic:** Must consist of at least 95 percent organic ingredients.

- **Made with organic ingredients:** Must contain ingredients that are at least 70 percent organic and 30 percent nonorganic. However, the 30 percent nonorganic may not be GMO.

There's no conclusive evidence showing foods classified as organic are any healthier than conventionally raised foods. Many consumers believe the flavor of organic foods is better than that of conventional products. Farming and ranching practices, the location of farm or ranch, and the length of storage of products can all affect a food's taste and nutritional content.

Products coming from small local farms and ranches have shorter transit and storage times; thus the flavors of these foods are fresher than those of some larger conventional producers and handlers. Sometimes these local farmers and handlers aren't certified through the USDA as organic due to the expense and time involved. They may have organic practices, but they cannot legally claim their products are organic.

Prices generally reflect the added expenses farmers and ranchers incur from certification and practices. These expenses are passed onto consumers in the form of higher prices. When you make the decision whether organic produce is right for you, you must also take into account the perceived benefits with the cost. If you find you want to purchase organic but simply don't have the budget to match your desire, consider starting with organic versions of produce on the Dirty Dozen list of foods with the highest content of pesticides.

 WAKE-UP CALL

The Dirty Dozen refers to the top 12 fruits and vegetables you may want to consider purchasing as organic. The Environmental Working Group (EWG) is a nonprofit, independent group that conducts random pesticide residue testing on fruits and vegetables. Over two thirds of the samples of produce on this list tested positive for pesticide residue.

The Dirty Dozen includes the following, with two additional items I've added added to the end of the list:

- Apples
- Peaches
- Nectarines
- Celery
- Cherry tomatoes
- Cucumbers
- Grapes

- Potatoes
- Snap peas
- Spinach
- Strawberries
- Sweet bell peppers
- + Hot peppers
- + Kale and collard greens

Although the previous produce items tested positive for the most pesticide residue, they still fall within acceptable ranges based on governmental guidelines. The following list called the Clean Fifteen lists produce that tested the lowest in amounts of pesticide residue:

- Asparagus
- Avocados
- Cabbages
- Cantaloupes
- Cauliflower
- Eggplant
- Grapefruit
- Kiwis

- Mangoes
- Onions
- Papayas
- Pineapples
- Sweet corn
- Frozen sweet peas
- Sweet potatoes

Certification Process

Created in 2002, the USDA Organic Seal has become the standard of excellence for organic products. The seal's standards specify how crops and livestock should be raised. It's easy to find this seal on a variety of products throughout your local grocery store. No matter where in the world the products come from, if they carry the USDA Organic Seal, the producer or handler has passed a certification process. Producers and handlers must participate in a yearly onsite review to ensure that the USDA standards are being met. Produce also undergoes random periodic residue testing. California has its own specific set of standards, which allows additional regulations for products produced within that state.

When you see the USDA Organic Seal on a product, you can be assured the product has been verified as following specific standards. There are three categories under the USDA organic standards:

- **Organic crops:** Must not use pesticides that are prohibited, GMOs, irradiation, material from wastewater, and manmade fertilizers.

- **Organic livestock:** Must have access to the outdoors and their handler must provide 100 percent organic feed and meet all animal health and welfare standards. Animals may not receive antibiotics or hormones to promote growth.

- **Organic multi-ingredient foods:** Must be composed of at least 95 percent certified organic components.

Land that has been farmed with conventional methods must undergo a period of 36 months where products that are prohibited for organic use are not applied to the current crops grown. After that 36-month window, then the products may be certified organic.

The producer or handler must describe their operation in writing, which includes listing all products they'll produce or raise. A history of all substances applied to the land in the previous 36 months must also be provided. In addition, they must write an *Organic System Plan*, which includes the practices they'll follow to ensure all standards are met.

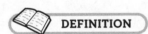 **DEFINITION**

An **Organic System Plan,** also called the Farm Plan, is a system of practices that helps farms plan ahead for problems and situations beyond their control. By having this plan in place, farms are able to forecast sales and expenses, assisting them in maintaining economic viability. Producers and growers are also better equipped to look at their natural resources and see how they can best utilize and conserve them.

Costs to the producer or handler vary depending on the size and type of their operation and the products produced. Certification costs can range from a few hundred to several thousand dollars. There are also yearly fees to maintain their certification as well as a sales tax on their products.

After the application and fees have been submitted, an certifying agent ensures the applicant's practices are in compliance with the standards and an inspector conducts an onsite evaluation. If all facets comply with the USDA standards, the certifying agent issues the organic certification.

From this point, the certification is reassessed on an annual basis. Documentation must be provided and inspections must also be carried out. The certifying agent again reviews documents and completed inspection reports to determine if standards are consistently being met to maintain organic status.

Natural Ingredients

The term "natural" is one of the most misused and misunderstood terms in food labeling. Any food that's processed in any way is no longer technically natural. There actually is no legal definition for "natural." However, the FDA has stated products may also be defined as natural if they don't have additional color or ingredients that are manmade or contain artificial flavors. In 1990, the USDA Food Safety and Inspection Services (FSIS) published a rule clarifying what may constitute natural on food labels with regards to poultry and meats.

Natural flavors may consist of spices, spice extracts, essential oils, and oleoresins. According to the USDA, products with an animal origin, such as dried broth or meat and meat extract, may not be labeled as having "natural flavoring" or "flavoring." Proteins from natural sources that have undergone a hydrolyzation process also may not be labeled as natural. These products must be labeled as hydrolyzed and include the source of the protein, such as "hydrolyzed milk protein" on the label.

 FOODIE FACTOID

Oleoresins are considered an allowed natural additive to foods. They're comprised of a combination of essential oils (oleo-) and a semisolid portion of plants or trees (-resin). These products are extracted from plants, such as herbs and spices, and trees like pines and birches.

Beyond the previously specifications listed, the term "natural" should mean nothing to consumers. Be cautious when choosing one product over another claiming it's natural. The best approach is to read the ingredient list and make the decision for yourself.

Genetically Modified Organisms (GMOs)

GMOs are currently in hot debate. GMOs are organisms whose DNA has been altered, meaning selected genes from one organism are inserted into the DNA of another organism. The intent is to change or enhance a certain behavior or attribute.

Recombinant DNA, in the form of genetic engineering, has been around since the early 1970s. GMOs have been used extensively in pharmaceuticals, biological and medical research, gene therapy, and agriculture. Insulin is an example of the success of GMO in the pharmaceutical industry. Food from GMOs is called *GM food*.

Attributes of GM foods are generally deemed as favorable to the supply chain, and ultimately, the consumer. Often, the use of genetic engineering increases the food supply and lowers the food's price. GM foods may have a longer shelf life, be easier to transport, and be pest resistant.

Many GM crops are designed with the intent to resist disease and pests or be protected against weed killers. According to the World Health Organization (WHO), the ability to create a crop with bacteria resistant to herbicides has resulted in less herbicides being applied.

Many consumers question the safety of GM food. According to WHO, foods are deemed safe when they have been in our food supply for decades without causing illness or disease. The new GM foods are rigorously studied under strict standards to ensure safety for the environment and human health. These same standards are not upheld for conventional foods.

The safety of GM foods is critical, and the need for testing is widely accepted. Standards for testing GM foods include testing for toxicity, potential allergens, toxins, nutritional benefits, side effects due to the gene insertion, and the stability of said gene. Because GM food is created in different ways by varying technology, each food needs to be tested and considered individually. All GM food products currently on the market have passed all safety testing.

Food Additives

Food additives are either man-made or natural. They are products added to a food that doesn't contain said additive in the food's original form. Additives are classified as either direct or natural.

Direct additives are often added to foods during the production process. These additives make the end product more appealing to consumers. Natural additives are include spices, vinegar for pickling, and salt for curing.

According to the National Institute of Medicine (NIM), food additives may be used to enhance nutrition, improve texture, maintain freshness, control the acid-base balance, or enhance flavor and nutrition.

Additives are not always a negative addition. The USDA has compiled a list of additives that are Generally Recognized as Safe (GRAS). Potential allergies and sensitivities aren't accounted for under the GRAS guidelines. There are close to 400 additives on the list, including salt, caffeine, calcium citrate, ascorbic acid, and agar.

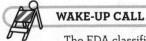 **WAKE-UP CALL**

The FDA classifies monosodium glutamate (MSG) as a flavor enhancer and foods containing this additive must be labeled. While listed on the FDA's GRAS list, many feel they experience an adverse reaction to foods in which it's used. According to the Mayo Clinic, no scientific evidence has been found to show a relationship between symptoms and MSG. Any reaction is likely to be short term. If a reaction is experienced, it's recommended to avoid foods containing it in the future.

Additives on the GRAS list are classified using a numbering system from 1 to 5. Items categorized as 1 have no evidence demonstrating the potential of harm. An additive classified as a 5 on the scale means there's a complete lack of studies to determine whether it is safe or unsafe. Less than 5 percent of additives are classified as a 5.

> **NOTABLE INSIGHT**
>
> When determining the safety of food additives, the NIM states the legal definition of "safe" as defined by Congress: "Safe" is the "reasonable certainty that no harm will result from use."

What Is a Sustainable Food System?

Healthy and sustainable are completely different facets of food. Foods may be sustainable without being healthy. Organic farming practices are generally sustainable agriculturally. However, organic products may be shipped across the country, affecting the carbon footprint and thus their true sustainability.

Consumers should be cautioned about products using words that imply sustainability. Phrases such as "cage-free," "free range," or "natural" do not have legal definitions and may not actually be sustainable practices.

Locally Grown

The term "locally grown" generally refers to food products raised or grown within a range of 150 miles around the end user. Often consumers get confused by multiple messages, such as "locally grown," "organic," and "sustainable." Products may incorporate all three labels; however, each is a component on its own and they aren't interchangeable.

Local sourcing is becoming more popular with restaurants and retail food outlets. Consumers are requesting locally grown and produced items, which keeps the money spent in the community and helps the local economy. Local sourcing also means smaller quantities can be purchased due to decreases in transportation cost and time. Food items are fresher with less exposure to the possibility of time and temperature abuse. Often with local sourcing, the "middle men" are eliminated. The consumer purchases directly from the source, thus decreasing the time from producer to end user.

NOTABLE INSIGHT

According to Seafood Watch, sustainable seafood refers to fish and seafood caught or farmed in ways that don't negatively impact the environment. Fishermen and fisheries have incorporated sustainable practices to ensure the viability of the individual species for future generations. Look for the Marine Stewardship Council (MSC) ecolabel when shopping or ordering fresh seafood. This label ensures your selection comes from a source that has undergone a certification process and is reviewed for its sustainability practices.

The availability of products year-round is one of the biggest obstacles to overcome when considering local sourcing. Most of the country is not able to produce or raise comparable food products in the off months as they do during prime weather conditions. Purchasers must have back-up options for purchasing in case local providers are not able to meet their needs.

Environmental Impact

The impact of the products we consume on our environment is also considered from the producer all the way down the line to the final consumer. Many businesses have incorporated practices of reducing their carbon footprint in exchange for slightly higher prices. Individuals in charge of purchasing are making the effort to choose products that have low or zero levels of toxins, a reduction in pollutants and fragrances, are more energy efficient, and in general promote the health and welfare of their employees and consumers.

Fresh, Frozen, Canned, or Freeze-Dried?

Fresh produce is generally best when it's affordable. Packed full of vitamins, minerals, and fiber, fresh produce is key to a healthy diet. Eating a variety of colors ensures you get a wide array of nutrients to keep you as healthy as possible. Check your cart when you shop to ensure your food selections match the colors of the rainbow.

When stocking up on fresh fruits and vegetables, plan to use varieties likely to spoil quicker at the beginning of the week, such as berries and leafy greens. Produce such as apples, carrots, and potatoes have a longer shelf life and prices stay fairly stable. Premixed salad bags are quick shortcuts, keep fairly well, and are prewashed.

Potatoes get a bad rap because of their high glycemic index and carb count. But in reality, one russet potato contains about 150 calories and is loaded with potassium. Potatoes are inexpensive, have a long shelf life, and are easy to cook for a speedy dinner.

Purchase assorted snack-size veggies to eat on the go. Carrots, celery, cucumbers, broccoli, and bell peppers are all great choices to have on hand. These versatile vegetables keep fairly well and are easy to bag up for snacks.

Buy fruits like melons, peaches, plums, grapes, and berries when they're in season. Fresh fruit can be expensive, but consider the health benefits and put the cost into perspective. Are you willing to pay $4 for a hot latte but not for a pint of blueberries?

The produce section is filled with convenience foods to make it easy to eat healthy on the go. Check out the produce cooler for bags of apple slices, fresh fruit cups, and sliced melon. There are also precut veggie cups and mixed veggie trays of various sizes. Try precut peppers, onions, and fresh mixed stir-fry vegetables to make cooking super simple. For on-the-go snacks, grab single-serve veggie and dip packs or a premade salad.

Frozen fruits and vegetables are picked at their peak of freshness, making frozen produce a wonderful option. Items can be kept in your freezer for months and pulled out when you've eaten up your fresh purchases. Look for varieties without sauces and added seasoning or butter. Frozen fruits and vegetables are also great in smoothies, stir-fries, and soups.

Canned varieties are processed more than fresh or frozen. However, the canned vegetable aisle has good products and better products. Choose vegetables, including beans, that are reduced sodium or no salt-added varieties. It's a good idea to rinse canned vegetables and beans under cool water before cooking to wash away more of the sodium. Look for varieties without added sauces and seasoning.

Canned fruit can also be a good option if it's chosen wisely. Fresh or frozen fruits are preferred over canned for their nutritional content. However, if it means you otherwise won't be eating any fruit, canned is acceptable. Canned fruit should be packed in its own juice. Avoid those sold packed in syrup or with added sugar.

 WAKE-UP CALL

Canned food may seem as though it would last forever. However, sometimes a can's contents will interact with the metal and cause a chemical reaction to occur. According to the University of Minnesota Extension, rust can occur, causing small holes not seen by the naked eye. Acidic items, such tomato sauce, will corrode the can, resulting in a change in quality, taste, and nutrient content. Temperatures above 100°F also can alter the food's nutrient content and risk spoilage.

Freeze-dried fruits and vegetables offer another version of produce. The American Institute for Cancer Research (AICR) recommends freeze-dried fruits and vegetables as a healthy alternative to fresh. One serving (¼ cup) can pack almost as much of a nutrition punch as a serving in its original form. These freeze-dried versions are filled with phytochemicals, vitamins, and minerals. Nutrients that are susceptible to heat, such as vitamin C, are not as plentiful. The lightweight versions also lack the water content found in other fresh produce.

Truth in Labeling

As previously discussed, the FDA regulates and enforces labeling on foods. In 1994, the Dietary Supplement Health and Education Act was passed. This act deregulated the supplement industry. Currently, supplements sold in the United States don't need to be approved before going on the market. The FDA requires manufacturers to follow good manufacturing practices (GMP). The FDA only reacts to complaints and doesn't approve or authorize products.

Independent certification services can perform audits to ensure supplements have the nutrients in the amounts specified and no additional ingredients are contained in the product. Private certification agencies include ConsumerLab, NSF, and USP. Not having a private audit doesn't necessarily mean the product isn't safe. The same concept applies to those with the seal of certification—not all testing is foolproof. Choose the supplements you take wisely.

The Least You Need to Know

- Understanding your food's supply chain can help you make the best food choices.
- Always read the food label to learn what's in your food, where it comes from, and if there are any additional ingredients such as food additives or flavor enhancers.
- Recently harvested produce will always be more flavorful. Seek out local farms or farmer markets in your area for a healthy variety of foods and to help your local economy.

Cooking Oil Basics

Every kitchen should be stocked with good-quality cooking oils. The type of oil you use most often should be a healthier variety, such as olive or canola oil, which are better for heart health.

There are many types of oils available in the marketplace today, and selecting the right ones can be confusing. Another factor in choosing the appropriate oil is how you'll use it in your recipes. In this chapter, we'll discuss the assortment of fats used in cooking oils and the best ones for the job and for your health.

In This Chapter

- Discovering the best oils for a healthy heart
- How long can cooking oils be kept?
- The role of trans fats in the food industry
- Saturated fats and their negative impact on health

Choosing the Right Cooking Oil

There are a variety of reasons people use certain oils to cook with. For some it may be about the flavor, for others ease of use; some may have heard a certain oil is heart healthy, as in the case of olive oil. Others may use a certain type or brand of oil because that's what was used in the household in which they grew up. Whatever the case, it's important to examine the predominant type of oils in your diet.

Cooking oils are 100 percent fat, provide about 150 calories per tablespoon, and are made up of fatty acids. Each fatty acid is divided into a different category based on their molecular structure. The three categories are saturated; unsaturated, which includes monounsaturated and polyunsaturated; and trans fatty acid—or as it's commonly referred to, trans fat.

Saturated fat comes from animal products such as dairy, red meat, and poultry. It's referred to as "bad" fat and is solid at room temperature. Saturated fat means there are hydrogen atoms attached to each carbon atom, thus the atoms are saturated with hydrogen.

Research has shown that saturated fats adversely affect blood lipid levels by increasing your cholesterol and LDL, which can increase your risk of cardiovascular disease and type 2 diabetes. Butter and lard are saturated fats commonly used in cooking.

Monounsaturated and polyunsaturated fats are typically liquid at room temperature. Monounsaturated fats like olive oil will partially solidify when refrigerated, whereas a cold temperature will not affect a polyunsaturated fat like canola oil.

Monounsaturated fats are commonly referred to as heart healthy, and their association with good health came about from findings based on the Seven Countries Study in the 1960s. In this study, the main source of fat found in the people's diet was olive oil, and the study gave rise to what we now refer to as the Mediterranean diet.

Polyunsaturated fats can also be beneficial to your health, as they posses the same ability to lower cholesterol levels when consumed in moderation. Polyunsaturated fats include omega-3 and omega-6 fatty acids.

The trans fat in our diets is not found in nature, and has been chemically altered in a lab. It's actually worse for you than saturated fat, and is solid at room temperature. Research from the Harvard School of Public Heath reports that consumption of just 2 percent of calories from trans fat daily equates to a 23 percent increase in the risk of heart disease.

Oils can be costly, and they don't have a long shelf life once opened. It's also important to purchase the right volume amount for your household use. It's not wise to purchase 2 gallons of oil at your local big-box store because it's cheaper when there are only two of you in your household. A good-quality extra virgin olive oil will only last from 3 months to 2 years unopened in a cool, dark pantry.

Rancid oil is easy to identify by its putrid smell. Many report it has a "paint thinner" smell. When oil becomes rancid, it has been oxidized and aldehydes have formed, causing the varnish- or paintlike smell.

 FOODIE FACTOID

> A UC Davis study had subjects taste 22 extra virgin olive oils. Researchers were surprised to learn that 44 percent of the participants preferred the taste of rancid oil opposed to the bitter and pungent flavors in high-quality extra virgin olive oils.

When selecting the primary oil you'll use for cooking, you need to understand the pros and cons of each type to make an informed choice. You must consider flavor, use, smoke point, and health needs. Most people should have two or three oils on hand in their kitchen.

The Best Monounsaturated Oils for Health

Monounsaturated oils are better for your heart. Consumption of monounsaturated fats helps decrease total cholesterol levels and LDL (bad) cholesterol, and increase HDL (good) cholesterol. They also help lower blood pressure, and the oil is a source of vitamin E. The following list shows the percentage of monounsaturated fats in common cooking oils.

- Macadamia nut oil: 84%

- Hazelnut oil: 82%

- Safflower oil: 79%

- Olive oil: 78%

- Avocado oil: 65%

- Flaxseed oil: 65%

- Canola oil: 62%

- Peanut oil: 48%

- Sesame oil: 41%

The most commonly used and researched monounsaturated oil is olive oil. Spain produces most olive oil and has about 5 million acres, compared to California at 30,000 acres. Spain takes an average of 6 months to harvest and California has only a 2-month harvest window, according to the North American Olive Oil Association.

Olive Oil

Olive oil is a very versatile, heart-healthy oil. It's made from the pressing of the whole olive, including the pit. It takes about 10 pounds of olives to make 4 cups of oil.

The olive-producing countries have an established set of standards to distinguish between the types of oil, such as extra virgin and refined. The International Olive Oil Council provides one set of guidelines.

In 2008, California passed a law regulating labeling requirements for olive oil. The U.S. government developed standards for grades of olive oil in 2010, but it's voluntary for producers.

Each type of olive oil is graded and labeled accordingly, based on the characteristic of the oil. Generally, the higher quality the oil, the lower the acidity.

FOODIE FACTOID

The four enemies of olive oil are time, temperature, oxygen, and light. The amount of time it takes to get the fruit from the tree to the press needs to be minimal. The temperature needs to be held constant, and you must minimize exposure of the oil to heat and cold. Oxygen accelerates the oxidation process and speeds up rancidity, so oils must be tightly bottled. Light can cause damage from UV rays, which is why oils are packaged in tinted bottles to protect them from light.

Olive oils vary greatly in flavor and aroma. There are three key flavor profiles in olive oil: fruity, bitter, and pungent. Fruity is described as buttery, floral, grassy, green, nutty, apple, artichoke, and herbaceous. Bitter is simply bitter tasting, which is a good thing. It typically means there's a higher antioxidant content in the oil. Pungent oil has a peppery taste, and may slightly burn the back of your throat as you swallow it.

There are several types of olive oil available in the marketplace, including extra virgin, virgin, ordinary virgin, pure, refined, and light-tasting olive oil. Extra virgin makes up about 60 percent of all sales. Let's take a look at the key types.

U.S. extra virgin olive oil is derived from the first cold pressing of olives. The oil is extracted without added heat. Although the pressing action itself causes friction and thus heat, temperatures are maintained and are not allowed to exceed 85°F. The oil is then collected, filtered, and bottled. Due to this process, extra virgin contains the highest amount of phytochemicals. It also has the strongest flavor with the lowest acidity level and no defects. It has a smoke point of 325 to 375°F. You can cook with extra virgin olive oil, but just don't exceed the smoke point, as you'll negate many of the beneficial health properties within the oil.

U.S. virgin olive oil has a few defects as compared to extra virgin and still has no heat applied during processing. It has a good flavor as opposed to an excellent flavor in extra virgin.

U.S. olive oil is a blend of refined and virgin oils. It's flavorless and odorless. The refining method does not alter the chemical structure of the fat. Vitamin E oil can be added back into the product to make up for what was lost during production. It has a smoke point of 465°F.

U.S. olive pomace oil is a blend of olive pomace oil and virgin olive oil. It's extracted from the leftovers of the fruit and pits along with an added chemical solvent and applied heat. It's the lowest grade of olive oil you can purchase. The flavor is very different from extra virgin oil and may taste flat. It has a smoke point of 460°F.

When shopping for olive oil, it's important to identify the following:

- What's the country of origin where the olives were grown?

- How fresh is the olive oil in the bottle? What's the harvest date?

- How was the bottle cared for? Is it in a store window with the sun shining on it or is it outside at a farmers market?

- What seals are on the bottle? Does it have seals of certification from the following sources: COOC-certified extra virgin olive oil, Non-GMO, or Kosher?

Canola Oil

Canola oil was originally derived from the rapeseed plant, which has been bred naturally into what we now call the canola plant. Canola oil is extracted from the seeds of the plant. A pod develops from the flower that resembles a pea pod, but is much smaller with about 20 black-brown seeds. The seeds are crushed and the oil is extracted and refined.

Canola oil is a pale golden color with a very neutral taste. It has a smoke point of 400°F. It makes a great choice to use in a salad dressing or emulsification, such as in mayonnaise when you don't want to impart a flavor. It's also a good option for baked goods and for use in frying.

Research reported in the *British Journal of Nutrition* showed that in subjects with high cholesterol levels, the consumption of canola oil instead of flaxseed oil help to lower their LDL cholesterol and total cholesterol levels. Another study published in the *Journal of Internal Medicine* replaced dietary fat with canola oil and showed a decrease in triglycerides in subjects with high cholesterol levels, along with an overall improvement in serum lipoproteins.

Avocado Oil

Avocado oil is made from the pulp or flesh of the avocado. The avocado's flesh can contain 30 percent oil, which is bright green in color due to high levels of *chlorophyll* and carotenoids.

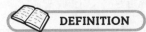

DEFINITION

Chlorophyll is a green plant pigment. It allows a plant to capture light energy and convert it into plant energy through photosynthesis.

Avocado oil extraction is similar to olive oil extraction in that it's cold pressed without any added solvents; however, water and enzymes can be used.

The mild flavor of avocado oil has been described as having a hint of avocado taste along with a slight butter and mushroom flavor. It can be used in any recipe without imparting any off flavor. Furthermore, it has an extremely high smoke point, between 480 and 500°F, depending on whether it's cold pressed or refined, which makes it great for frying or using on the grill.

Limited research exists on avocado oil, as it's a fairly recent newcomer to the marketplace. One study reported in the *Journal of Periodontal Disease* states that it reduced inflammation in those with periodontal disease. Avocado oil is higher than olive oil in monounsaturated fatty acids, so it makes sense to expect that it offers the same heart-healthy benefits as olive oil.

Safflower Oil

Safflower oil is extracted from the seeds of a thistlelike annual plant grown in the western Great Plains region in the United States. The plant produces yellow, orange, and red flowers, and it's allowed to dry in the farmer's field prior to harvest.

The seeds are then harvested from the flower and are classified as monounsaturated or polyunsaturated. They are sent to processing plants to extract the oil. The monounsaturated oil is used for cooking. The polyunsaturated oil is used in cold applications, because it's not shelf-stable and must be refrigerated.

Safflower oil is just 1 percent higher in monounsaturated fatty acids than olive oil, and its taste is very mild. This oil can be used in a variety of recipes from baked goods to sautéing and frying, since it has a very high smoke point of 450 to 510°F depending on how refined the product is.

FOODIE FACTOID

The petals of the safflower blossom can be used as a substitute for saffron, the most expensive spice in the world, which comes from the crocus flower. In the center of each flower are three stigmas (strands) of saffron.

Polyunsaturated Oils

Polyunsaturated fats are essential fats in your diet. A polyunsaturated fatty acid has two or more double bonds in its carbon chain. The chains are classified as omega-3 or omega-6. Both omega-3 and omega-6 are beneficial to your health. Research has shown that replacing saturated fats or highly refined carbohydrates with polyunsaturated fats reduces LDL levels in the blood along with triglycerides, and improves the overall cholesterol profile.

Omega-3

The highest amounts of omega-3s are found in flaxseed. However, walnuts, canola oil, and soybean oil also contain omega-3s.

Flaxseeds come from the flax plant, which grows in cool climates. Flaxseed oil is golden yellow in color and has a nutty flavor. It should not be heated higher than 120°F, so it's not recommended to cook with. However, it can be great to add to foods after the cooking process.

Flaxseed is approximately 57 percent alpha-linoleic acid (ALA), which is an omega-3. Much research has shown positive effects of diets high in ALA in relation to cardiovascular disease. The Nurses' Health Study involving 76,763 women revealed that women who consumed less ALA in their diets had a higher risk of sudden cardiac death. Studies have also looked at the protective effects against inflammatory disorders such as rheumatoid arthritis, as well as improved immune function in people with lupus.

A review of the research showed that it also lowered cholesterol levels in postmenopausal women and in people with high cholesterol levels.

Omega-6

Corn, safflower, soybean, walnut, and sunflower oils are high in omega-6 fatty acids (linoleic). Omega-6 is an essential fatty acid. Research has shown omega-6s may help alleviate pain associated with diabetic neuropathy, improve insulin resistance in diabetics, and decrease blood pressure. Other studies examined the role of omega-6 in children with attention deficit hyperactivity disorder (ADHD), which reported a reduction in overall symptoms.

Americans consume a higher ratio of omega-6 to omega-3 in their diets, which can inhibit the benefits of omega-3. Ideally, you need to work toward a 1:1 ratio. Most omega-6s come from processed foods. Let's take a look at common oils high in omega-6s.

Soybean Oil

To make soybean oil, the beans are split open, heated, and pressed flat like rolled oats. Next a chemical solvent is used to extract the oil. It has a pale color and neutral flavor, and is a favorite in the food industry as an all-purpose oil. Additionally, the smoke point is 450°F, which makes it an excellent choice for frying. Soybean oil can also be used in any type of recipe, including baked goods and desserts.

Corn Oil

Corn oil is extracted from the germ of the seed. It's *expeller pressed* and a chemical solvent is applied. It also goes through a degumming and alkali treatment, winterization, and removal of waxes, and then finally steam distillation.

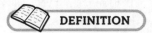 **DEFINITION**

Expeller pressed is a mechanical extraction process that applies pressure until the oil is released from the seeds. This method will render about 65 to 70 percent of the oil.

Corn oil has a pale yellow color and nutty taste with a hint of corn. It has a 450°F smoke point and is a good choice for high-heat applications like frying. Overall, it's a good neutral cooking oil that can be used in a variety of recipes.

A study published in the *Journal of Clinical Lipidology* showed a reduction in cholesterol and LDL through the use of corn oil when as compared with extra virgin olive oil. Another study showed that corn oil is high in phytosterols, and researchers believe it's the phytosterols that aid in cholesterol reduction as opposed to it being an unsaturated fatty acid.

The Negative Impact of Oils on Health

Saturated fats, when consumed in high amounts increase total cholesterol and LDL cholesterol levels in the blood, and overconsumption can increase your risk of heart disease and stroke. It may also increase your risk of type 2 diabetes. The American Heart Association (AMA) recommends no more than 6 percent of your total calories come from saturated fat.

Saturated fats predominantly come from animal sources. These fats are solid at room temperature, such as butter and lard, which are used in cooking. The fatty part around beef steaks, pork, and lamb is also a saturated fat.

Butter

Butter is a saturated fat that is made from churning fresh cream or milk. The butterfat is then separated out by the mechanical action. Butter is legally defined as being "made exclusively from milk or cream or both, with or without common salt, and with or without additional coloring matter, and containing not less than 80% by weight of milkfat."

European-style butters have more fat and less water. Some have additional bacterial cultures added to increase its sweetness and to add tanginess. European butter is churned longer than its American counterpart. The additional churning time decreases the water content, and thus increases the fat content to 84 percent to create a richer profile.

Butter is evaluated by USDA graders, produced in an approved plant, and comes in different grades. U.S. Grade AA is made from sweet fresh cream and has a sweet flavor and smooth, creamy texture. U.S. Grade A is also made from sweet fresh cream and has a smooth texture, but the flavor profile differs slightly from grade AA. The taste may seem a bit flat. U.S. Grade B butter is only sold in a few areas and has an acidic flavor.

Butter can be frozen and will maintain its quality for 2 months. It's sensitive to odors in the fridge, so be sure to keep it tightly covered. The best way to use butter is to let it sit out 10 to 15 minutes prior to use. Butter can be used in a variety of recipes from sauces to baked goods. Keep in mind that the smoke point of butter is 350°F.

 FOODIE FACTOID

It takes 5 gallons of whole milk to produce about 2 pounds of butter.

Lard

Lard is made from pork fat. It has 25 percent of the saturated fat of butter. Lard is known for making crispy piecrust and pastries. Lard creates flakier baked goods because it doesn't contain any water, and as the fat molecules in lard melt they create little air pockets or layers of flakiness in foods.

Most of the lard found in the marketplace has been hydrogenated to increase shelf life. However, some high-end butcher shops carry lard you can purchase and render down for use in cooking. Good-quality lard has a neutral flavor and a smoke point of 370°F, which makes it a good choice for frying and a favorite of Southern cooks.

Palm Oil

There are two types of oil made from the fruit of the palm tree, which grows in tropical regions like Malaysia and Indonesia. Palm kernel oil is made from the kernel or pit inside the fruit, and palm oil is made from the fruit pulp. Palm kernel oil has a negative impact on health and raises cholesterol levels. However, it's not sold as cooking oil, but is used for making soaps, detergents, and cosmetics.

Palm oil is similar to coconut oil in molecular structure. Palm oil is golden yellow in color, tasteless, and is predominantly used in the food industry. The smoke point of palm oil is 465°F.

Coconut Oil

Coconut oil is made from the flesh of the coconut by compressing it under high pressure. The mechanical extraction produces some heat, but the temperature doesn't exceed 120°F. There are no government standards for producing coconut oil. If the product refers to "virgin" oil, it typically refers to the fact that the oil has not been refined or bleached. Coconut oil has a mildly sweet flavor and velvety texture, and is great for sautéing foods as it imparts a subtle sweetness. It has a 350°F smoke point.

Coconut oil is a saturated fat and contains lauric acid, a medium-chain triglyceride. For many decades, coconut oil has been considered a "bad" fat because it is saturated. However, many avid fans of coconut oil tout it as being the cure-all to almost every health-related disease. Unfortunately, sufficient research doesn't exist to back up these claims.

A review of research in relation to heart disease and coconut oil includes found that people consuming coconut oil did see improvement in HDL, but it also increased their LDL. Another study comparing coconut oil, beef, and palm oil, reported that coconut oil raised their total cholesterol and HDL as compared to beef and palm oil. A large study of Filipino females reported high levels of HDL in those who had the highest intake of coconut oil.

In relation to weight loss, a small pilot study showed a significant reduction in waist circumference. A double-blind clinical trial in 2009 compared soybean oil to coconut oil in obese women and revealed no change in body weight, but did report a reduction in waist circumference in the group consuming coconut oil. Though it looks to be beneficial in relation to HDL, the increase in total cholesterol may negate the benefit. Additional research need to be done on coconut oil and the effects on lipid levels in the body. It's still a saturated fat and should not be consumed in large amounts in a healthy diet.

Trans Fat

Very little trans fats occur in nature. They're present in small amounts in butterfat, beef, and lamb, but it's a different molecular structure in nature than what is created in the lab. Trans fats are created when partially hydrogenated oils are chemically altered to add additional hydrogen molecules to make the liquid oil solid. In 2013, the U.S. Food and Drug Administration (FDA) deemed trans fatty acids as unsafe for use in human foods. Researchers began in the 1990s looking at the affect of trans fat in relation to heart disease and stroke. Research showed that trans fats actually increased LDL and lowered HDL.

The food industry liked using trans fats because they had a longer shelf life and were inexpensive. Commercial fryer oil is one example where trans fats were used in the restaurant industry. Additional sources in the diet are baked goods, snack foods, and stick margarines, although most margarine manufacturers have reformulated their products to make them trans fat-free. However, trans fats still exist in products even though the FDA no longer recognizes them as safe and they were removed from the Generally Recognized as Safe (GRAS) listing. The National Academy of Sciences states "trans fatty acids are not essential and provide no known benefit to human health." However, it's estimated that 5 to 8 percent of total calories consumed in the American diet are from trans fatty acids.

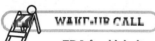

WAKE-UP CALL

FDA food labeling law allows food manufacturers the ability to list "0 grams" of trans fat on a food label even though it may actually contain a range of 0 to 0.5 grams. A look at the label will help you identify the trans fat by the words "partially hydrogenated oils."

Vegetable Shortening

The term "shortening" used to refer to lard or margarine, but nowadays shortening means a vegetable-based product. Shortening made prior to 2007 was hydrogenated and contained trans fats. Companies have reformulated their products to remove the trans fat, and these new formulations contain a little less than 1 gram of trans fat per serving.

Nonhydrogenated shortening can also be made from palm oil. It's semi-solid in texture, contains little water, and is shelf-stable. Vegetable shortening has a neutral flavor and can be used in baked goods such as biscuits and piecrusts. It can also be used to make cake icing. The smoke point of vegetable shortening is 360°F. Vegetable shortening is one of those fats you might have on hand during the holidays for baked goods, but it certainly is not for daily use.

Margarine

Margarine is made from a variety of monounsaturated, polyunsaturated, and saturated fatty acids from vegetable oils and animal fats. The more solid the form, the more saturated the product. When liquid oils are partially hydrogenated to solidify them, trans fat is formed. When selecting margarine, the spreadable tubs typically contain less trans fat than the sticks. However, it's important to read the label. The American Heart Association (AHA) recommends people shop for margarine with less than 2 grams of saturated fat per tablespoon.

 FOODIE FACTOID

Margarine was invented in 1869 by French chemist Hippolyte Mege-Mouries. It was made from beef tallow and called oleomargarine. *Oleo* is Latin for beef fat and *margarite* is Greek for pearl.

Margarine was intended to be a healthier option to butter when it hit the marketplace. Unfortunately, no one was aware of the trans fat issue and its detrimental effect on health. There are still many varieties available on store shelves, and you can use them in any recipes where you would use butter. Margarine's smoke point ranges between 302 and 320°F. It's important to taste the different brands to find a flavor profile you enjoy. Keep in mind that most margarine will still contain some trans fats, so it's important to read the label.

The Least You Need to Know

- Try tasting a variety of heart-healthy olive oils to find one that fits your flavor preferences.
- Purchase oils in small quantities to ensure they will be fresh and not go rancid before you get a chance to use them up.
- Seek out good sources of omega-3s and omega-6s for the beneficial health effects.
- Watch out for trans fat in food products you eat regularly by reading the ingredient list.

Your Healthy Diet

In this part, you'll learn what a healthy diet looks like and how to ensure you're getting the right portions. You'll discover that eating a variety of foods is key. You'll understand how to recognize your body's food cues and deal with food cravings. You'll learn how to tell the differences between a true food allergy, food intolerance, and food sensitivity. We'll also tour your kitchen and see how it measures up to get you cooking for optimum nutrition. We'll take you through the basics of organizing your kitchen and discuss the right foods to keep on hand.

We also realize that on occasion you'll want to dine out, so we'll show you how to navigate a restaurant menu, provide tips on making healthier selections, and how to eat out if you have allergies or sensitivities.

What Is a Healthy Diet?

A healthy diet has a different meaning to different people. Your view of what constitutes a healthy diet will change over time. When you make small changes that become new habits, you reset what your view of a healthy diet. A healthy diet is not about excluding foods. It's about variety, moderation, portion control, and including new healthy foods.

The World Health Organization (WHO) recommends starting healthy eating habits early in life. By maintaining a healthy diet throughout each phase of your life, you'll help prevent cancer, heart disease, diabetes, stroke, and other health problems.

In This Chapter

- The right blend of nutrients for a healthy diet
- How do your foods measure up to the standards?
- Dishing out more whole grains, fruits, and vegetables to build a better plate
- Favorite foods and your eating routines
- Food ruts and what to do about them

Meeting Your Body's Needs

Getting the nutrients your body needs from foods varies from person to person and from day to day. Age, sex, fitness, activity level, and disease effect how many nutrients your body requires on a daily basis.

What you ate in your twenties without gaining a pound probably won't work in your forties. Most people find they need fewer and fewer calories to maintain the same weight as in their early years.

Mixing up your diet and adjusting the amounts of carbohydrates, protein, and fats in the foods you eat is a good place to start. It's also important to listen to internal cues from your body and its messages regarding hunger, fatigue, and mood. This, along with regular exercise, will help you achieve optimum health.

Nutrients for Health

Your diet should contain a blend of carbohydrate, protein, and fat. When these energy components are combined, these three groups will total 100 percent of your calories. The Institute of Medicine (IOM) recommends certain percentage *acceptable macronutrient distribution ranges (AMDR)* that each component should contribute to your diet for optimal health.

Carbohydrates should comprise 45 to 65 percent of your calories daily. This equates to about 100 to 145 grams of carbohydrates daily, based on a 2,000-calorie diet. Carbohydrates generally come from starchy vegetables, fruits, and grains. Aim to make half of your grains whole grains.

Protein should comprise between 10 and 35 percent of your calories, or about 50 to 150 grams daily, based on a 2,000-calorie diet. Selecting a variety of lean protein sources is key. Choose from plant-based proteins (legumes, beans, nuts, and seeds) and animal protein (dairy, eggs, fish, lean chicken, and meat).

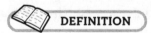 **DEFINITION**

A recommended percentage **acceptable macronutrient distribution range (AMDR)** for carbohydrates, proteins, and fats helps ensure people take in enough healthy nutrients in their diets while limiting others (such as fat) to help ward off disease. These standards are part of the Dietary Reference Intake and are determined by the IOM.

The AMDR for fats is 20 to 35 percent of your calories, which works out to 45 to 78 grams daily for a 2,000-calorie diet. WHO recommends fat should not exceed 30 percent of the total calories consumed. In addition, they recommend replacing saturated fats with unsaturated fats (poly- and monounsaturated). Following the WHO recommendations, your fat intake should not exceed 67g per day.

Added sugar is any sugar added during the processing or formulation of foods. It doesn't include sugar that occurs naturally in foods, such as in fruits and vegetables. Sugar is added to soda, baked goods, protein bars, salad dressings, and ketchup just to name just a few. WHO recommends added sugar should not be more than 10 percent of the total calories consumed. For a 2,000-calorie diet, this equals no more than 50g per day (or less than 12 teaspoons per day). One teaspoon of sugar contains 4.2 grams of fat. The U.S. Department of Agriculture (USDA) reports that excessive added sugar intake can lead to increased triglyceride levels and weight gain, which are precursors to various other diseases.

Salt or sodium is another component of foods most Americans get too much of. The recommendation from the USDA is 2,300mg per day, and the average American consumes close to 5,000mg per day. Some foods are a natural source of sodium, such as celery and eggs. However, most of the sodium we consume comes from prepared and processed foods. Foods high in sodium are generally low in potassium, which has an opposite effect on blood pressure than sodium. WHO recommends increasing potassium intake from fresh fruits and vegetables and decreasing sodium-laden foods.

Determining how much of the three energy components are in your diet can be tricky. New technology, such as online, tablet, and smartphone apps, can come in handy. Many apps and web-based programs do the work for you by breaking down what you eat into graphic charts that display your overall calorie distribution. These apps can track the distribution daily and provide you weekly and monthly averages.

Food labels are a quick and easy way to estimate percentages by simply looking at the percent daily values (%DV), which are based on a 2,000-calorie diet. The downside is not every meal will have a food label attached to it. Determining the proportion of these three components on your plate by using labels can be time-consuming. A simpler approach to estimating your meal makeup is to simply look at your plate.

Here's how to rate your plate.

1. Look at your plate and determine what portion are carbohydrates (grains, bread, fruit, yogurt, milk, starchy vegetables, and added sugar). It should be about 50 percent.

2. Estimate your serving of proteins (animal products, grains, beans/legumes, and dairy). It should be about 20 to 30 percent.

3. Identify sources of fat (oils you eat and cook with; salad dressings, dips, and condiments; fat in protein, cheese, eggs, dairy, nuts, and seeds). It should constitute less than 30 percent.

Some of the foods in these categories overlap. You may be able to count one food in two groups. For example, dairy is a good source of carbohydrate and protein. As you can see, this could get quite complicated. By utilizing online programs or apps to track your foods, you can get a clear picture of the breakdown of each energy nutrient. This will help you to decrease or increase quantities to create a more balanced diet.

Variety

Variety is important to keeping yourself on a healthy track. Eating the same things day after day becomes monotonous and lessens your joy in life.

Think of the nutrients as an all-you-can-eat buffet. If every time you only eat two things, you'll miss out on everything else. Choosing different items of varying colors (red, orange, yellow/white, green, and blue/purple) will ensure you get a variety of antioxidants, vitamins, and minerals. Look in your shopping cart and ask yourself, "Do my selections match the colors of the rainbow?"

It's important to vary your protein selections, too. If you only eat chicken, you miss out on the omega-3 fatty acids in fish. If you skip eggs, you may be lacking in biotin. Grains contain different types of fiber, amino acids, and vitamins. *Quinoa* is considered a complete protein—it contains all essential amino acids in sufficient quantities. However, there's even a difference between the red and white varieties. Oats are high in soluble fiber, and wheat is high is phosphorus.

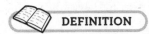 **DEFINITION**

Quinoa is an ancient grain originally harvested by the Incans in Peru. There are over 100 different varieties of quinoa, but we mostly see red and white in our grocery stores. Red quinoa has a slightly different nutrient profile than white, but both are good sources of protein, fiber, B vitamins, iron, magnesium, phosphorus, and zinc. Try it as a substitute for rice in your next meal.

If you eat the same foods cooked the same way every day, can you taste them any longer? Eating a variety of foods helps to reinforce mindful eating. Trying new foods will lead to new taste adventures and help ensure you get all the nutrients you need.

Portion Control

The term "serving" is open to interpretation. Your idea of what a serving of pasta is will be completely different from everyone else's version. Most serving sizes are much larger than what is actually considered a nutritional serving. Rethinking serving sizes is the first place to start when you're working on portion control. Use measuring cups to measure out portions for a few weeks until you learn what a serving size looks like on your plate, in your bowl, or in your glass.

Have you ever considered how the size of your plate affects your portions? A dinner plate should be approximately 8 or 9 inches in diameter. If your plate is larger, consider using a salad plate for your meals or purchasing smaller plates. When serving your plate, fill half of it with vegetables and fruits, and divide the remaining half between whole grains and lean proteins with dairy on the side. This method can help keep you in check when you eat out.

Another good idea is to plate your food in the kitchen rather than serving family-style at the table. Be sure to put leftovers away so you aren't tempted to get up from the table for seconds. Replace empty-calorie beverages with milk or milk alternatives and water at mealtimes.

Eating meals and snacks throughout the day will help you manage your portion sizes, and you'll be less likely to overeat. If you notice your weight is creeping back up, it might be a good idea to recheck your portion sizes and bring out those measuring cups.

Serving Size Tips and Techniques

Here's a quick guide to help you determine what an actual serving size is.

- 1 cup vegetables (the size of a small fist)
- 2 cups leafy vegetables
- 1 cup fruit or a small piece (the size of a tennis ball)
- $1/4$ cup dried fruit
- $1/3$ cup rice, pasta, barley, or quinoa
- $1/2$ cup cooked oatmeal
- 1 cup milk
- 8 ounces yogurt
- 1 ounce cheese (1-inch cube)
- $1/4$ cup nuts and seeds (fits into the palm of your hand)
- 1 tablespoon oil, nut butter, hummus, or salad dressing (the size of the top half of your thumb)
- 4 ounces fish, meat, or poultry (the size of a deck of cards)
- 1 large egg

Practice these tips every day for a week and portion control will be a snap.

SERVING SIZE TIPS AND TECHNIQUES

Here is a quick guide to help you determine what an actual serving is.

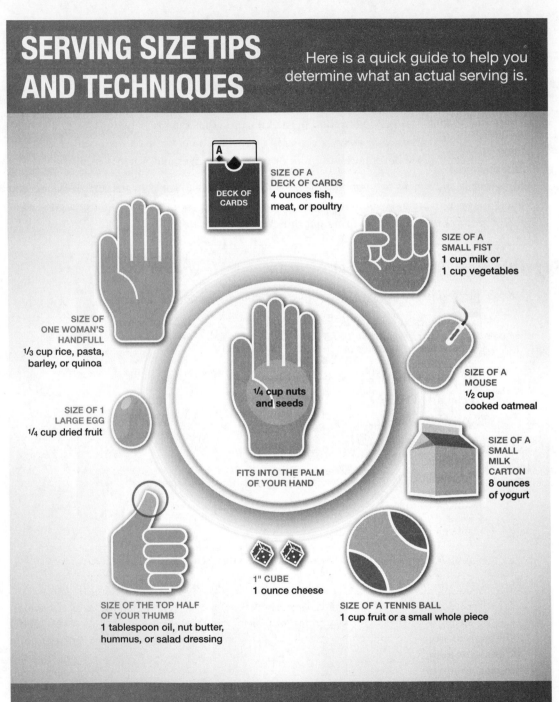

DECK OF CARDS

SIZE OF A DECK OF CARDS
4 ounces fish, meat, or poultry

SIZE OF A SMALL FIST
1 cup milk or 1 cup vegetables

SIZE OF ONE WOMAN'S HANDFULL
1/3 cup rice, pasta, barley, or quinoa

SIZE OF A MOUSE
1/2 cup cooked oatmeal

SIZE OF 1 LARGE EGG
1/4 cup dried fruit

1/4 cup nuts and seeds

FITS INTO THE PALM OF YOUR HAND

SIZE OF A SMALL MILK CARTON
8 ounces of yogurt

SIZE OF THE TOP HALF OF YOUR THUMB
1 tablespoon oil, nut butter, hummus, or salad dressing

1" CUBE
1 ounce cheese

SIZE OF A TENNIS BALL
1 cup fruit or a small whole piece

Practice these tips every day for a week and portion control will be a snap.

Gadgets

There are some essential tools for getting a handle on portion size. A good set of dry and liquid measuring cups to measure out servings will help you get the hang of what a cup of milk or ⅓ cup of rice looks like. Another good investment is a kitchen scale that weighs in both grams and ounces. It should also be able to be zeroed out when you put an empty bowl on it. Using a kitchen scale will help you learn exactly what 4 ounces of chicken or a 125-gram apple looks like. An inexpensive scale runs about $20.

If cooking meals quickly is imperative, consider microwave-cooking devices such as a microwave steamer. You can steam vegetables and fish and reheat whole grains in a snap. If you're cooking for one, consider purchasing a toaster oven. You can broil or poach fish and chicken, roast vegetables, and toast nuts, all without turning on your main oven.

Your Food Nemesis

You're not alone in your food cravings. A study from the Research Center on Aging at Tufts University showed over 90 percent of women experienced food cravings. Foods eliciting strong cravings tended to be high in fat and calories and low in fiber and protein. Research showed reducing portion size had the largest impact on their long-term body mass index (BMI). In addition, those successful with weight loss didn't give in to their food cravings as frequently as those with less weight loss.

A study published in *Appetite* reports researchers have found a link between carbohydrate intake and *serotonin* release. During meals and snacks high in carbohydrate and low in protein, large amounts of insulin are released, which lowers your blood sugar. This allows an easier passage for the amino acid tryptophan to head to the brain and make serotonin. Protein blocks the effect and mediates the release.

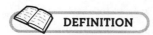

DEFINITION

Serotonin is a chemical in the body that acts as a neurotransmitter. It's made from the amino acid tryptophan. Most of the serotonin is found in cells in the GI tract. Small amounts are made and used in the brain. When released, it produces feelings of happiness and a sense of well-being. Serotonin deficiencies may cause depression, mood and sleep disorders, and sexual dysfunctions. There are ways you may be able to boost your levels of serotonin. Exercise and alteration in thoughts and diet have shown positive results.

Researchers at the University of San Francisco report a relationship between stress and food cravings. Certain regions of the brain are activated during food cravings. Research shows the brain sends out signals correlating to craving fat and sugar. After ingesting fat and sugar, the brain has a reduction in stress hormones and is calmed. Carbohydrates get a bad rap for cravings because when they're consumed they release serotonin and help calm us down. However, most of the high-carb foods we crave also contain high amounts of fat. Think potato chips, ice cream, and cookies, for example.

A study reported in the *International Journal of Obesity* showed a correlation between the reduction of high-fat foods and feelings of anxiety and withdrawal. It's thought that completely eliminating high-fat foods may lead to an increase in food-motivated behavior.

Becoming self-actualized about your eating habits will help you overcome your food nemesis. Many times we have foods we simply can't resist. We know they're not the best choice to help us reach our health goals, and in fact they may actually be harming us. This nemesis is about more than just the food.

The first step in self-actualization about your eating habits is to identify your food nemesis. Is it the ice cream in the freezer calling to you at night? The pastry staring at you from the case as you wait in line for your morning cup of Joe? Often a food nemesis is habitual and we give in to it on a daily basis without really thinking about it. Before you can change the behavior, you need to stop and evaluate the emotional hold it has on you.

Food cravings can be triggered by emotional responses. Learning to deal with these responses in healthy ways will reduce these triggers. Tell yourself food will not help you feel less stressed or make you happier. Think of other ways you can feel better other than eating what you're craving.

An important factor in weight loss is to reduce the portion size of your food nemesis. When you decide it's time to give in, portion out the food. Use small bowls or bags to make your allotted portion seem bigger. Don't sit down with the entire bag of chips or container of ice cream. When you portion out the food, stop and look at it. Smell it and savor each bite. Be present in the moment. If your willpower is lacking and you find it difficult to keep your portion sizes smaller, then purchase single-size servings to have on hand for snacking.

Reducing the frequency of giving in to cravings is another key component to successful weight loss. One approach is to gradually wean yourself from it. Try limiting the food to every other day, then down to once a week, and eventually once a month. It's also a good idea to only purchase a single-size serving to help limit its impact on your diet. It also may be helpful to not purchase the item at all. If the food is not in the freezer or cupboard, you can't use it as a "go to" after a bad day of work.

For some people, changing to a low-fat or low-calorie version helps with the craving. Eating a low-fat brownie or ice cream satisfies the craving without jeopardizing the diet. However, always use caution with this method. Don't allow yourself to have larger portions to make up for the reduced calories.

How to Cultivate New Food Habits

Don't expect your food habits to change overnight. Make small changes a few at a time, and when those become habits, make a few more. Don't get discouraged. You'll have cravings, get sidetracked, and get stuck in a food rut from time to time. Keeping track of your progress can help your motivation.

The Plan

Good health doesn't just happen; you have to plan for it. Having healthy foods on hand will make the healthy choice the easiest choice. Pick a day to sit down and plan out meals for the week. Plan to have three meals a day with one or two snacks.

Understand your lifestyle and be realistic. If you work 12 hours a day, you know it's unrealistic to cook an elaborate dinner when you get home. If you find the lack of time is your biggest constraint, shop and prep foods on your day off. You can then precook proteins and grains, wash and cut up vegetables, and assemble lunch containers for the week to grab on your way out the door. Make yogurt parfaits, veggie and hummus combos, salads (with dressings on the side), sandwich kits, and heat-and-serve dinners. Seriously, nothing is better than coming home starved and opening the fridge to find a delicious dinner already made.

Avoiding and Dealing with Cravings and Ruts

"Why am I craving potato chips right now?" Ask yourself these questions the next time a craving sets in. Are you tired, overly hungry, or had a rough day? Or do you eat potato chips every day at lunch? Being honest with yourself as to why you have a food craving can be the first step in overcoming it. If the craving is mood-related, do something about the mood. If you're tired, take a nap, go to bed earlier, or sit quietly and relax for a few minutes. If you're lonely, reach out to a friend, take your dog to the park, or go on a walk.

Did something happen today you just can't shake? Try meditating quietly, writing in a journal, or making an action plan to resolve the problem. If your cravings are habitual, make a new habit. Have chips every day with lunch? Replace them with crunchy vegetables dipped in hummus and only have chips with your lunch on Fridays. Food will not resolve your problems.

We all get into food ruts. By being a creature of habit, you don't have to think and make decisions. You may order the same entrée, pack the same lunch, or eat the same breakfast. Maybe you stop for a latte every day on the way to work or celebrate Friday nights with pizza and beer. You may buy bananas, apples, and lettuce every time you go to the grocery store because it's easy.

Change won't happen by itself. Incorporate a new plan by looking at sale ads and buying fresh fruits and vegetables you might not have tried otherwise. Set a goal to try a new recipe once a week. Getting out of a rut will lead to more mindful eating. You'll actually start to think mindfully about what you're eating and spend time tasting foods rather than just shoveling them down.

Getting Sidetracked

We all get sidetracked. Old habits can be hard to break, even when we think we're past them. Vacations and holidays are often times we revert, make excuses, and give ourselves permission to eat unlimited amounts. It's okay to eat your grandma's stuffing at Thanksgiving, your mom's holiday cookies, or pizza at a famous restaurant while on vacation. Enjoy the splurges and move on. Good nutrition is not a sprint, it's a marathon.

The Least You Need to Know

- A healthy diet doesn't happen overnight. It requires a commitment and planning.
- Identifying correct food portions is a quick and easy way to manage your weight.
- Try new foods—you never know what you've been missing out on.
- Changing a lifetime of food habits is hard work, so be gentle with yourself and allow for setbacks.
- Practice mindful eating habits and don't let your emotions rule your food choices.

Hunger

Every day, your body requires food in order to function properly. How and when you fuel your body will affect your short-term performance and longevity. Your thoughts and practices involving food can be quite strong and may have taken years to form your routines or habits. Sometimes these old habits haven't been the best in relation to your health, and occasionally they can lead to serious health issues and eating disorders.

In this chapter, we'll discuss how your body communicates with you about food both in positive and negative ways using hunger and satiety cues. We'll also examine how people use food to deal with stress and emotions. You'll also learn about fad dieting and the physical and biochemical impact on the body.

In This Chapter

- How your body reacts to hunger
- Learning to recognize hunger and satiety cues
- What to eat to fight stress
- The harmful effects of fad diets
- Your emotional relationship with food

Hunger Regulation in the Body

Your body is designed to alert you when it needs food. It may try to communicate this to you by a feeling of light-headedness, a headache, nausea, an overall lack of concentration, or even stomach grumbles. Hunger is a complex process regulated through hormonal actions controlled by your brain.

The hypothalamus controls hunger and satiety in your body. The lateral hypothalamus controls hunger, and the ventromedial hypothalamus controls satiety. Research has shown that when the lateral hypothalamus is destroyed or damaged, it causes a lack of desire to eat or anorexia to occur. Conversely, when the ventromedial hypothalamus is damaged, it causes an uncontrollable urge to eat all the time. Hunger and satiety work together to provide the fuel and nutrients for your body to function properly.

The Physical Need for Food

We discussed a few of the physical symptoms associated with hunger, such as lightheadedness. However, your brain receives all sorts of neural data from your body on the status of blood sugar levels, hormones, circulating fats, and proteins that are used to control your desire to eat or not eat.

Your body needs to eat every 3 or 4 hours and especially after an all-night fast while you slept. Eating every three to four hours tells the body that there's a regular source of nearby nutrients. When the body doesn't get food regularly, it goes into starvation protection mode, which sets off a cascade of events and leads to weight gain.

After a refreshing night of sleep, you awake and your blood sugar levels will be toward the low end of the scale if you're healthy. A signal is then sent to your brain to report the need for energy. Your body may also be receiving a signal from your empty stomach. The epithelial cells located in your stomach release ghrelin, which is a hormone that stimulates appetite and leads to those physical hunger pangs. Ghrelin can be released in response to low blood sugar levels and high stress levels, too. Upon receiving a hunger signal from the body, most people would seek out food and eat. However, due to busy schedules we can override those helpful signals on occasion, which is not necessarily a good thing and can lead to a negative impact on your health.

As you eat, your stomach expands and the amount of ghrelin begins to decrease because the stomach is stretching and food is now present. Stretch receptors in the stomach also communicate back to the brain that food has been received and it's now satisfied so the hunger alert can subside.

NOTABLE INSIGHT

Researches at Yale performed a study in which they served college students two identical chocolate milkshakes on two separate occasions. However, participants were told that one shake was a high-calorie "indulgent" shake and the other was a low-calorie "health" shake. Blood levels revealed that ghrelin decreased when they consumed what they *believed* to be the decadent shake and ghrelin levels remained constant after consumption of the healthier shake. Researchers concluded that the hormone might be able to be altered by your mind-set.

As food is digested, absorbed nutrients are distributed throughout the body and bloodstream. The hormone cholecystokinin (CCK) is released to digest fat and protein, and it informs the brain that it's no longer hungry. The brain then senses these levels and can further inhibit hunger by increasing glucose levels.

Leptin is a hormone produced from fat cells in your body. It tells the brain that fat stores are low and you need more fat now. Once you eat and digest the fat, it gets stored away, which then causes the fat cells to secrete more leptin. The brain then recognizes the increased level of circulating leptin and tells you to stop eating. Leptin's primary role in the body is to help prevent starving or overeating in order to keep you alive and functioning.

When there's a problem with leptin (called leptin resistance), the body doesn't recognize the high circulating levels of leptin. It then also slaps us with a weight gain whammy by reducing our energy expenditure, placing us in the "conserve energy" mode, and burning fewer calories while at rest.

This is one reason why diets don't work—because as we lose body fat, the body is working behind the scenes in conservation mode to use less energy and replace the lost fat stores. Additionally, researchers believe leptin may actually compel us to eat and regain the weight that was lost. In people with leptin resistance, research has shown that it may be due to inflammation, elevated fat levels in the blood, and a high circulating level of leptin.

Stress can also instigate hunger. The body's normal reaction to stress is the fight or flight response, where your body gets pumped full of epinephrine (adrenaline) which allows you to get out of the way of whatever frightened you. Your appetite actually shuts down and blood is directed away from the digestive tract and into your extremities. Prolonged periods of stress can also cause another stress hormone, cortisol, to be released from the adrenal glands. Cortisol causes you to seek out foods to calm you down, such as those consisting of sugar and fat. This hormone also regulates other hormones like neuropeptide Y, leptin, and corticotrophin-releasing hormone (CRH), all of which act to stimulate appetite and lead to overeating and weight gain.

Some foods can help you negate stress. Complex carbohydrates such as warm oatmeal, warm milk, turkey, walnuts, dark chocolate, oranges, spinach, and fatty fish like salmon high in omega-3s can help even out those stress hormones. The physical act of chewing on crunchy foods like carrots and celery sticks can also have a calming effect. Stress is a part of modern life. You need to find a healthy way to deal with it, whether it be a combination of stress-fighting foods or regular exercise and meditation.

The Psychology of Hunger and Emotional Eating

As we discussed previously, your hormones play a big role in your response to hunger and satiety, but many other factors contribute, such as cultural influences, the social aspect of eating itself, and what you were taught as a child.

Growing up, you may have learned that you must clean your plate in order to have dessert, or perhaps food was used as a reward for good behavior. Whatever the case, those food rules stay with you and can be very difficult to change as an adult.

Your eating habits are affected by culture. The constant barrage of media depicting underweight males and females drive the public toward unrealistic weight goals. This leads to a mentality that you must be extremely thin in order to be likable and successful in today's society. These subliminal messages influence your eating habits and force you to make a choice of constant restriction with a feeling of "never being good enough" or overeating and a "screw it" attitude, both which lead to dysfunctional eating habits.

 FOODIE FACTOID

When visiting China, you should note the host will be embarrassed if food is not left on your plate or if there are not leftovers on the table, as it's a sign that the guests didn't get enough to eat.

The social aspect of eating affects how and what you eat. For instance, men and women generally eat less in the presence of the opposite sex. Everyone tends to eat more or less depending on the actions of others in the group. In a study in *The American Journal of Clinical Nutrition,* obese children were paired with friends who were also obese. They were allowed to eat as many snack foods as they wanted. The results showed that the children consumed an additional 300 calories as opposed to when the obese children were paired with strangers.

Body image also has a huge influence on your eating habits. Your body image is your mental picture of your body, which is a completely subjective image. You can have a negative or positive body image. It's usually influenced by the reactions of others about one's body and self-observation. Your body image includes aspects such as weight, height, shape, how you *feel* in your body, and what you believe about your appearance. A person's body image can influence several aspects of their life. For example, it can impact our mental and physical health, and how we treat ourselves. Body image can also influence how we relate to and interact with other people.

A negative body image can be described as having a distorted perception of size and shape, and it can develop from various external influences. It comprises feelings of being uncomfortable, awkward, ashamed, self-conscious, and anxious. In Western culture today, a big factor in perceiving your body image is the media. Women are idealized for their petite figures and men for their sculpted muscles. It can be hard to deal with constant reminders of your body size if idealistic bodies appear on social media, television, billboards, the internet, and in magazines. Other influences include frequent comparison to others, abuse, prejudice/discrimination, and negative comments from other people.

The most severe form of negative body image is referred to as body dysmorphic disorder (BDD). Individuals with this disorder become obsessed with their perceived flaws. BDD can adversely create problems in work, school, and relationships with friends or family. It can also cause depression, anxiety, or thoughts of suicide. Although serious, there is treatment for BDD with a combination of psychological therapy and medication.

Positive body image is a true and clear perception of your body's shape and size. You can enjoy your body because you're proud and appreciative, and accept your body the way it is. People with a positive body image know that bodies come in all shapes and sizes. They can determine value and character without the influence of physical appearance. Having a positive body image means your self-esteem is not affected by your weight or height. Everyone has their own assessments of their body.

Disordered Eating Patterns

Disordered eating differs from diagnosed eating disorders like anorexia nervosa because the symptoms are less frequent and less severe. The Academy of Eating Disorders defines disordered eating as "when food and eating create psychological pain and suffering." However, it still puts a person at a greater risk of the behavior developing into a true eating disorder. When a person's social life is adversely affected by the inability to eat with friends or family due to avoidance of certain foods or if the event conflicts with exercising, there is need for concern.

 NOTABLE INSIGHT

The National Association of Anorexia Nervosa and Associated Disorders state that 1 out of 10 people diagnosed with eating disorders is male. Males tend to be overlooked by family members and health professionals, which can lead to serious health issues due to delayed treatment.

As with all dysfunctional eating, it's simply not just about the food. There's a deep underlying cause that must be dealt with for the person to have a healthy relationship with food. If the person is unable to move away from these disruptive patterns, it may be necessary to seek professional help.

Examples of disordered eating patterns are:

- Preoccupation with and avoidance of certain foods
- Strong sense of self-esteem attached to body image
- Chronic yo-yo dieting
- A strict and excessive exercise regimen
- Use of purging or laxatives to maintain weight
- Compulsive or emotionally driven eating

Eating Disorders

The primary types of eating disorders are anorexia nervosa, bulimia, binge-eating disorder, and disorders not otherwise specified. It's estimated by the National Eating Disorder Association that over 10 million Americans—men and women—experience an eating disorder in their lifetime. All of these disorders involve an unhealthy relationship with food, abnormal self-body image, and low self-esteem, along with extreme control and manipulation of weight.

Eating disorders are complex and involve genetics, metabolism, and psychological and social issues. Certain eating practices can trigger or intensify an eating disorder. Skipping meals, religious fasting, cleansing types of diets, and excessive calorie counting can all be triggers in people predisposed to an eating disorder. Each will require a combination of therapies to rebuild a healthy relationship with food.

Where to Find Help

Eating disorders require a multifaceted approach, which may involve psychological and/or nutritional counseling, and prescribed medications, because it isn't really about just the food or weight. People suffering from an eating disorder may require admission to an in-patient facility with 24-hour monitoring, depending on the severity of the disorder. Most can be treated through outpatient settings and support groups.

If you suspect someone may have an eating disorder, keep in mind that you can't just force a new way of eating on them and make it all better. However, you can be supportive and encourage them seek help to deal with the problem.

To locate treatment centers, practitioners, and/or a support group in your area, contact the following organizations:

National Association of Anorexia Nervosa and Associated Disorders: 630-577-1330 from 9 A.M. TO 5 P.M. CST Monday through Friday or email anadhelp@anad.org

Overeaters anonymous: www.oa.org

 NOTABLE INSIGHT

Approximately 45 million Americans go on a diet each year, with the majority being women.

Why Diets Don't Work

With each new year there's the birth of a new fad diet that's been popularized by the media or a celebrity. These diets typically focus on eating or the avoidance of certain types of foods like the cabbage soup diet, the grapefruit diet, the baby food diet, and the lemonade diet. They typically suggest you can lose 5 to 10 pounds in a week and they always sound too good to be true.

Regardless of the kind of diet, you'll lose weight on any diet when you alter your normal eating habits. The bad news is these short-term unhealthy diets can do more damage and make future weight loss even more difficult than it already is.

Most fad diets are extremely low calorie, which will negatively impact your metabolism as your body transitions into starvation mode. Additionally, it will become more efficient at utilizing calories, so your metabolism will slow down. As with any low-calorie diet, the scale will drop a couple of pounds daily, but this is typically due to water loss.

Short-term low-calorie diets typically have a diuretic affect. People believe they're losing body fat, which keeps them motivated to remain on the diet. Keep in mind that approximately 3,500 calories equals 1 pound of body fat. As your body stays on this low-calorie plan, you can bet the diet is nutritionally inadequate in a variety of essential nutrients. This will lead to alterations in cell metabolism, and it may not be able to prevent free radical oxidization. Therefore, the diet may actually be increasing inflammation in your body, which is not a good thing.

 NOTABLE INSIGHT

If quick-fix fad diets actually worked, the weight loss industry profits wouldn't be in the billions and the majority of the population would be skinny.

Protein is metabolically active, meaning your muscles burn calories. When you're on a very low-calorie diet, you're not taking in those essential amino acids. You're forcing your body to digest its very own muscle tissue to use for various body processes. You have essentially further reduced your energy-burning capacity while your body is at rest by lowering your basal metabolic rate.

Additionally, following these extreme fad diets for extended periods of time can also cause:

- Cardiac stress

- A decreased sex drive

- Depression

- Fatigue

- Hair loss

- Heart palpitations

- Irritability

- Sagging skin/increased wrinkles

- Shortness of breath

- A weakened immune system

There are no magic formulas when it comes to weight loss. You didn't gain the weight overnight; therefore you shouldn't expect it to come off that quickly. A sensible, healthy approach to eating that includes whole foods along with regular exercise is the only long-term solution.

One reason people often gain back weight after losing it may be related to the set point theory. This theory suggests that everyone has a predetermined weight the body wants to maintain. This theory was developed from research performed in 1982. The body's desire to maintain this "set point" is attained by increasing hunger, using fewer calories, and storing more fat. This point may be preset due to genetics, disease, stress, and dieting.

The set point is the body fat's thermostat. The theory suggests that despite your efforts to control your weight, the body will gravitate toward its set point. Your body has a 10- to 20-pound range at any given time that it feels comfortable at and will fluctuate between. This range is set to help your body maintain optimal functionality. Your body will fight to regain weight if you fall under your set point by conserving energy in ways such as slowing down metabolism and decreasing body temperature. Conversely, if you begin to exceed your weight's set point, your body will increase its metabolic rate and body temperature in an attempt to burn extra calories. The only thing that seems to lower the set point is regular sustained exercise over time.

Breaking Free from Old Eating Patterns

The first step in changing any type of pattern or habit is to acknowledge that it exists. Once it's acknowledged, you can make a conscious decision to change the behavior. Next, it's important to determine why you do what you do. Do you find that you follow a certain pattern because it's what you learned as a child, or is there another underlying cause? Whatever the case, you need to explore your feelings associated with the behavior you want to change.

Once you've determined what you want to change, you need to establish small steps to make the change possible. For example, let's say you've decided you would like to increase your servings of vegetables from one to five per day because it will help you lose weight by replacing higher-calorie items you are eating. It will also provide you with essential nutrients you were missing out on like phytonutrients, vitamins, minerals, and fiber. These are a few of the steps you might take toward this goal:

1. Identify one new vegetable you want to eat this week.

2. Determine where you'll purchase it.

3. Select a mealtime in which you want to include it.

4. Decide on a recipe to prepare it.

5. Eat and enjoy your new vegetable.

6. Determine if you'd like to eat more of this vegetable and how frequently you could work it into your meals each week.

7. The following week, add an additional new vegetable and begin the inclusion steps again.

Many people may think if one vegetable is good, then more is better. It is; however, it's much easier to incorporate small changes over time in order to developing healthier long-term eating habits. Keep in mind it takes about a month to change a habit and periods of stress can interrupt your progress and make you fall back on old routines. Don't despair; just start again, because one day of not-so-healthy eating won't negate a month's worth of healthy eating habits.

 NOTABLE INSIGHT

In 1925, the Lucky Strike cigarette campaign suggested one way to get slim was to grab a smoke instead of eating something sweet. Of course, back then the negative health effects of smoking were not known.

Clean Plate Club

Have you ever observed a friend or family member who will not let you remove his or her plate from the table until every scrap of food is eaten? This is what is referred to as the "clean plate club," which is a learned habit. Ironically, this originally started as a government campaign by President Woodrow Wilson in 1917. President Wilson created the U.S. Food Administration to help ensure that food staples didn't go to waste.

A study by Cornell University reports that the average adult eats 92 percent of everything on his or her plate. The same study also looked at meals eaten by males and females across seven different countries, and the results were the same: if it's on the plate, it was eaten!

Be a Good Role Model

Children are ever watchful of adults and model all their behaviors after adults. The best thing you can do if you have children is to help them develop good eating habits that will last a lifetime. Studies have consistently shown that a large percentage of obese children will grow up to become obese adults.

Try to involve children in the whole process when it comes to food, from shopping to preparing and cleanup, based on age appropriateness. At the table, children should be able to chose what to eat and how much. Make sure you offer appropriate size portions based on their age. The American Pediatrics Association suggests you follow these golden rules of eating:

1. **Divide responsibilities.** Allow children to choose what to eat and how much to eat.

2. **Teach your children to notice natural body cues for hunger and fullness.** Eat when you're hungry, and stop when you're full.

3. **Don't make children clean their plates.** There should never be any pressure associated with eating

4. **Eat together as a family.** Use this time to model the eating behavior you want to see in your child.

I'm Not Hungry

Going without breakfast is a learned habit that's hard to change, but you can gradually work in a small balanced meal of protein, fat, and fiber (complex carbohydrates). Remember, your body has been fasting for 6 to 8 hours, and it needs nutrients to get going and function at its best. Try waiting an hour or two after you wake up and then have a hot beverage like coffee or tea. Select a small amount of oatmeal with dried fruit and nuts, a little bit of yogurt and granola, or even an ounce of cheese with high-fiber crackers for your morning meal. Each of these options provides fiber, protein, and a fat to fuel your body for the morning.

This meal will help you be a little more alert and think more clearly, and you also won't be so ravenous when lunchtime comes. You'll automatically eat less because you aren't trying to compensate for a missed meal.

In 2013, a study from the Harvard School of Public Health found that men who skipped breakfast tended to eat more at night and also had a 27% higher risk of heart attack and coronary heart disease. In the 2010 *American Journal of Clinical Nutrition,* a study found that people who skipped breakfast as children and on into adulthood had increased levels of LDL and total cholesterol when compared to regular breakfast eaters.

If you don't already eat breakfast, it's time to start. Remember, it's best to take small steps in order to change a behavior. You'll be healthier in the long run.

 WAKE-UP CALL

> Europeans eat their largest meal at lunch, as opposed to Americans who have it at dinner. This may be part of the reason why Europeans have lower obesity rates when compared to Americans.

Eating on a Schedule

Regularly scheduled meals throughout the day can help you feel better, lose weight, and think more clearly. It's a good idea to have breakfast, lunch, dinner, and two snacks between meals depending on your schedule. Doing so will help your body know it's going to get fed and food isn't a scarcity, so there will be no need for it to go into starvation mode. It will also help you eat less at each meal because you won't be overly hungry. You might also find you're much more productive because you're more mentally alert and feel much better. However, don't get stuck eating at the exact same time of day. Check in with your body and listen to its hunger cues. It will tell you when it's physically hungry.

Intuitive Eating

Intuitive eating is a mind/body approach toward foods. It's about developing a healthy relationship with food and learning the differences between the physical need for food and emotional ones. Intuitive eating follows these basic principles:

- Eat when you're physically hungry.

- Stop eating when you feel full.

- Focus on the food you eat, along with the taste and sensations associated with it.

- Eat slowly and in a relaxed environment.

- Eat foods you enjoy.

- Acknowledge your feelings (tired, needing comfort, irritated) and don't use food to soothe your emotions.

- Exercise regularly.

- Resist labeling food as "good" or "bad."

- Don't diet.

One key tool that intuitive eaters use is to evaluate their hunger level by using a hunger scale. Rate your hunger on a scale of 1 to 10 and see where you are before your next meal. These are merely suggestions of how you may feel, so I encourage you to devise a scale of your own.

 WAKE-UP CALL

Research has shown in studies on twins that those who dieted were two to three times more likely to become overweight than their twin who did not diet.

The Hunger Scale 1-10

1: Starving, famished, weak, irritable.

2: Extremely hungry, hunger pangs, tummy grumbling.

3: Hungry—ready to eat now!

4: Still a little hungry and able to eat a bit more.

5: Neutral—not really hungry anymore but could eat more. Distracted from eating the meal.

6: Sense of fullness in stomach, slowing down, feeling of satiety.

7: Really full—ate one bite too many!

8: Uncomfortably full—need to unbutton my pants!

9: Painfully full—stomach hurts and I've got to go find the sofa and digest all this food for the rest of the day.

10: Overly full—you're ready to vomit.

A good rule is to never let your hunger go below a 3. Try to eat at a 3 when you're hungry and stop when you're full at a 6. You should be hungry between meals if you're listening to your body. Pay attention to what your body is telling you and respond to it appropriately.

Another tool you may want to use is a food log to help monitor your eating habits. In a food log you can also record the times you ate, the foods you consumed, your hunger scale readings, and your emotional state of calmness, stress, tiredness, etc., all associated with that particular mealtime. Journaling your meals in a food log will help illuminate any areas you need to work on and will show you if you use foods to deal with emotional states. Food logs can be the old-school style of pen and paper, or they can be kept electronically through apps you can find online. Food logs can be a great help towards making healthier food choices.

Satisfying Foods

Everyone has a certain meal they feel really "sticks to your ribs" and fills them up after a hard day's work. As it turns out, certain foods are actually more satisfying. The more satisfied you are, the less you'll eat. It's important that you take the time to think about what foods will satisfy your physical hunger based on your taste preferences. The following list will help you get started.

Satisfying Foods

- Apples
- Baked, broiled, and steamed potatoes with the skins on
- Beans and legumes
- Dried plums
- Eggs
- Hot soup
- Lean proteins like chicken, beef, pork, and lamb
- Nuts
- Oatmeal
- Popcorn
- Salmon
- Yogurt

Food Cravings

Everyone gets food cravings now and then. They can be triggered by an emotion, a biochemical change in the body, or by the season of the year. It's okay to seek out and enjoy those foods on occasion. The problem is that when you restrict yourself from having any of these foods, it will lead to overeating when you do get your hands on them. One way to deal with food cravings is to acknowledge the request, then wait a couple of hours and see how you feel. Do you still need that particular food, or can you wait and purchase it later in the week? The good news is that you only need a small portion to satisfy that craving, as research has shown your taste acuity declines rapidly after the first few bites.

FOODIE FACTOID

During pregnancy, women have strong food cravings and many crave nonfood items such as dirt, cornstarch, and ice. The eating of nonfood items is called *pica*. Eating dirt, which commonly occurs in the Deep South and also African countries, is typically associated with low iron levels in the blood of residents of those areas.

The Least You Need to Know

- Be kind to yourself and your body by never going too long without eating between meals.
- Get out of the "diet" mentality and choose to eat healthy foods you enjoy.
- Intuitive eating is part of the mind/body connection to food.
- There are no magic formulas for weight loss. You must create a personalized plan to eat healthier.
- Listen to your body's hunger and satiety cues, and eat by following the cues.

Food Allergies

A true food allergy can be seriously life threatening, which can make eating a little scary sometimes, especially when it involves children. Many people believe they're allergic to a certain food when in reality they merely have an intolerance or sensitivity to that specific food. The difference is that a food sensitivity or intolerance won't produce a reaction that could be deadly.

In this chapter, we'll take a look at the real differences between a true food allergy and a food intolerance or sensitivity. We'll discuss what it means to live with such issues, and how you can still eat healthy and enjoy food outings with family and friends.

In This Chapter

- The difference between food allergies, intolerances, and sensitivities
- The eight top allergens that plague American children and adults
- Live-threatening food allergies
- How you can learn to eat out and enjoy life with food afflictions

What Is a Food Allergy?

A true food allergy is when the body mistakes certain food proteins as harmful invaders and mounts an immunologic attack by producing antibodies, histamines, and other defensive mechanisms. The immune system attacks the proteins or other molecules in food after that food is digested and absorbed into the bloodstream.

Food allergies will always involve antibodies, but they may not always produce symptoms. When they do, it's called an *asymptomatic allergy.* When a person produces antibodies and has symptoms, it's known as a *symptomatic allergy.* In either case, food allergies can only be determined by testing for antibodies. A specific food allergy can be determined by eating, touching, or inhaling that particular food, which will cause your immune system to overreact. For example, if you have a peanut allergy, your body's immune system will recognize peanuts as intruders and will over-compensate by generating antibodies known as Immunoglobulin E (IgE). These IgE antibodies are directed to initiate a chemical release within certain cells, which then produces an allergic reaction.

Allergic reactions can be mild, such as sneezing or hives, or they can pose a greater risk by causing *anaphylaxis,* which requires immediate medical action. Most individuals with severe food allergies must carry a device called an EpiPen, which contains epinephrine, to counteract anaphylaxis. In an emergency, the epinephrine is injected into the thigh of the individual going into anaphylactic shock. Without the epinephrine, their throat may swell up and actually cut off air passageways, leading to death. Other less serious symptoms that may result from an allergic reaction include itchy eyes, throat, or nose; wheezing; congestion; skin rash; abdominal pain; vomiting; and diarrhea.

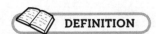 **DEFINITION**

> **Anaphylaxis** is a severe and life-threatening reaction that affects the whole body. The onset of anaphylaxis can happen within minutes or even seconds after exposure to an allergen. The chemicals released in response to the allergen can cause a person to go into shock. Blood pressure will drop suddenly and airways can narrow, making it difficult to breathe.

When a food protein is seen as a threat by the immune system, the body takes action but symptoms may not always occur instantly. Symptoms may be immediate or occur up to 24 hours after the food's consumption. If a reaction occurs immediately, it's easier to recognize which food caused the reaction. However, if that food caused a delayed reaction and symptoms don't appear until a day later, it can be challenging to identify because other foods have been consumed during that timeframe.

How do you determine which allergen caused a reaction? Determining a food allergy requires a physical examination, a complete health history, and diagnostic allergy testing. One of the most common tests for food allergies is the IgE skin-prick test, which uses food extracts to determine an allergic reaction. Usually a minimal amount of the specific allergen is injected into the skin with a small needle prick. If the area that was pricked becomes swollen or resembles a mosquito bite, it's recorded as a positive result for that specific allergen. This test is safe and effective and is usually done by an allergist, a physician who specializes in allergies and immunology. When a skin test isn't possible, an IgE blood test can also be performed to check the blood for certain antibodies to determine if there's a food allergy.

NOTABLE INSIGHT

True food allergies are not all that common. A majority of people who classify themselves as having a food allergy are really experiencing a food intolerance or sensitivity. The percentage of people in the United States who believe they have a food allergy is about 15 percent. However, the actual number of people who *do* have food allergies is about 3 to 4 percent. If you feel you have issues with a specific food(s), it's important to see your doctor to determine the real cause so it can be treated properly.

What Is a Food Intolerance?

A food intolerance occurs when there's a reaction to a food, but it doesn't involve an immune system response as with a true food allergy. It's often referred to as a non-IgE allergy. Instead, a digestive system response occurs when the person consumes a food that the gastrointestinal tract (GI) is unable to properly digest or break down. Reactions normally occur soon after ingestion, and can include gastrointestinal symptoms such as gas, cramps, bloating, nausea, stomach pain, vomiting, diarrhea, and heartburn. Other non-GI symptoms can also occur, such as headaches.

Many factors can contribute to a specific food intolerance. They can be caused by the lack of a specific enzyme such as lactase in lactose intolerance; or the culprit can be an intolerance to a certain chemical ingredient in foods such as added food coloring or sulfites. People with lactose intolerance can't tolerate any type of milk-related foods or beverages because they lack enough of the enzyme lactase, which is responsible for helping break down the milk sugar lactose. When lactose is not broken down properly, the result is usually GI upset. Keep in mind that this is *not* a milk allergy but an intolerance, which is very different. Examples of other less common intolerances include fructose and gluten intolerances.

Food intolerances can sometimes be difficult to diagnose. However, they usually can be discovered through trial and error to pinpoint which food is causing the symptoms. An elimination diet is helpful in uncovering the culprit, as well as a blood test and/or skin prick test to rule out a food allergy.

> **NOTABLE INSIGHT**
>
> Some people can experience an oral allergy syndrome, which is an allergic reaction to fruits and vegetables. People who have hay fever or are allergic to ragweed are more susceptible to this syndrome. Certain fruits and vegetables can cause tingling, itching, or swelling of the lips, tongue, and throat as well as itchy eyes, runny nose, and sneezing. If you find you suffer from this, pinpoint the foods that cause the reaction and avoid them. It definitely doesn't mean *all* fruits and vegetables will cause a reaction, so avoid those that do and continue to include other fruits and vegetables in your daily diet.

What Is a Food Sensitivity?

How do food allergies and food intolerances differ from food sensitivities? A food sensitivity is a non-IgE allergic response like a food intolerance. The difference is that food sensitivities do have an immune response. Unlike food intolerances, sensitivities can affect more than just the GI tract. Symptoms can include acid reflux, nausea, abdominal cramps, diarrhea, headaches, joint pain, fatigue, and a whole host of other issues.

Unlike allergies and intolerances, food sensitivities are often difficult to identify without testing because reactions can be delayed up to several days and can be dose-dependent, meaning an individual can sometimes tolerate a certain amount of the food causing the sensitivity. With food sensitivities, someone may consume a food with no apparent symptoms and then sporadically show signs of acid reflux, headaches, nausea, abdominal cramps, and other issues without being able to figure out why. This makes diagnosing specific food sensitivities pretty difficult. Tools such as an oral food challenge or trial elimination diet are often used to diagnose this issue.

A well-known food sensitivity that most of us have heard about is gluten sensitivity, which includes celiac disease and non-celiac gluten sensitivity (NCGS). This is not a gluten intolerance but a gluten sensitivity. Many Americans experience food sensitivities, and many of these sensitivities can be the result of another disorder, such as irritable bowel syndrome (IBS), inflammatory bowel disease (IBD), celiac disease, acid reflux, obesity, migraines, and many other conditions related to the foods we eat.

Lifestyle Eating and Performance

One definitive way to find out whether you're suffering with food sensitivities that may be causing chronic health problems is called a Mediator Release Test (MRT). An MRT is a simple blood test that measures your immune reaction or sensitivity to a whole host of foods, food additives, and chemicals. The MRT eliminates the guesswork by measuring delayed hypersensitivity responses to 150 different foods and chemicals.

This type of testing can often help identify culprits that a person cannot figure out any other way. The "hub" of the immune system is the gut. When people consume a food that are sensitivity to, the immune system sends out chemical mediators, such as histamine, cytokines, and prostaglandins, which can produce damaging effects to body tissues and cause the development of a wide array of symptoms and other major health issues. The MRT can help identify the possible foods that are triggering IBS, migraines, fibromyalgia, and other chronic health conditions. Depending on the types of mediators released, different areas of the body are affected. For example, for some people consuming a particular food will cause migraines, yet for others it may cause arthritis or acid reflux.

Identifying the harmful substance(s) is only the first step toward improving symptoms and issues. Once foods and/or substances are identified, the next step involves following an individualized Lifestyle Eating and Performance (LEAP) eating plan. To do this, you must work closely with your health-care practitioner and a registered dietitian nutritionist (RDN) who is LEAP certified. It's an effective protocol that combines the patented MRT with the skills of a certified LEAP therapist to produce a patient-specific diet. This specific diet plan identifies a list of safe foods to eat so that symptom improvement can begin immediately. Most individuals quickly overcome symptoms once the sensitivity is identified and the cause is eliminated. Many patients have been able to successfully eliminate chronic health problems within two to four weeks.

 NOTABLE INSIGHT

You can speak with your doctor concerning LEAP therapy and MRT testing or visit nowleap.com. Many therapists will counsel via phone, so you don't need to even reside in the same area.

The Top Eight Food Allergies

Known as the Big 8 or the top eight food allergens, the allergies associated with these allergens account for 90 percent of all food-related allergic reactions, and include wheat, eggs, fish, shellfish, dairy, peanuts, tree nuts, and soy.

To help Americans who suffer from food allergies, the FDA passed the Food Allergen Labeling and Consumer Protection Act of 2004 (FALCPA), which applies to all foods regulated by the FDA. This law requires food manufacturers to clearly label and identify in simple terms all eight major food allergens, or any protein derived from these foods, including any common names and their food sources. For example, if a label lists "starch," it must also specify whether or not the starch was made from or contains any wheat. As a result, food labels can now help consumers with allergies identify offending foods more easily so they can avoid them.

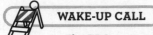

WAKE-UP CALL

The FDA estimates that anaphylaxis from food results in 30,000 emergency room visits, 2,000 hospitalizations, and 150 deaths annually.

Wheat

A wheat allergy is not the same thing as gluten intolerance or celiac disease. With celiac disease, the lining of the small intestine is damaged when any food with gluten (including wheat) is consumed, causing a host of symptoms and serious medical issues. With a wheat allergy, antibodies are produced in response to the consumption of wheat-containing foods. The protein found in wheat causes the immune system to overact and triggers an allergic response. Wheat allergies are most common in children and many outgrow it by age 3, according to the Food Allergy Research and Education organization.

A wheat allergy can be challenging as there are so many food products and beverages that contain hidden sources of wheat, such as beer, ketchup, and soy sauce, just to name a few. A wheat-free diet can include other whole grains that don't contain wheat, such as corn, oats, quinoa, rice, barley, and amaranth. If you're allergic to wheat, you're not necessarily allergic to all grains, only to the ones that contain wheat and wheat products. Just because a grain isn't labeled as wheat doesn't mean it doesn't contain wheat, so check *all* food labels and do your research.

Grains that contain wheat include:

Bulgur	Seitan
Couscous	Semolina
Durum	Spelt
Einkorn	Triticale
Farina	Wheat berries
Kamut	Wheat grass

Dairy

A dairy allergy is most commonly found in infants and children. According to Food Allergy Research and Education, it's estimated that about 2.5 percent of children younger than 3 years of age are allergic to milk. Reactions to a dairy allergy can include hives, wheezing, vomiting, diarrhea, abdominal pain, watery eyes, or a skin rash around the mouth. People who have an allergy to cow's milk may also react to milk from other animals like goats, as the protein in their milk is similar to that found in cow's milk. However, allergy testing is the best way to determine what can or cannot be tolerated.

Note that an allergy to milk is not the same as lactose intolerance. When a food allergy to milk occurs, the immune system reacts to the milk's protein by producing an allergic response. People who have lactose intolerance are simply missing a key enzyme that breaks down lactose. There's no immunologic response in people who are lactose intolerant; they just are unable to digest the milk protein, which normally causes GI symptoms. While these symptoms are uncomfortable, lactose intolerance is not life-threatening nor an allergy.

WAKE-UP CALL

If you have food allergies, it's vital to avoid cross-contamination. Anything you use, such as a toaster, cutting board, mixing spoon, etc., that may come in contact with an allergen should be thoroughly cleaned before being used for a nonallergen food. Avoiding cross-contamination can save you from having an allergic reaction.

Sources of milk can include:

Casein

Diacetyl

Ghee

Half-and-half

Lactalbumin

Lactoferrin

Lactose

Lactulose

Rennet casein

Sour milk solids

Whey

Fish

About 40 percent of people with a fish allergy experience the onset as an adult and usually have the allergy for life. Finned fish, including tuna, salmon, and halibut, are the most common fish allergens.

Most people who have a fish allergy are also allergic to more than one type of finned fish, so many physicians recommend avoiding all finned fish varieties. If you have a fish allergy, you need to always check food labels and ingredients lists for fish ingredients.

When a finned fish is cooked, its proteins are released in steam and become airborne. If you have an allergy to finned fish, it's advised to stay away from an area where fish is being cooked. Be extra careful if you do choose to visit a seafood restaurant. Even though you're not having fish, your nonfish meal could food be easily cross-contaminated by fish products. Symptoms include sneezing, hives, skin rash, headaches, or even anaphylaxis.

Unexpected sources of fish ingredients can include:

BBQ sauce

Bouillabaisse

Caesar and other salad dressings

Imitation fish or shellfish

Worcestershire sauce

Shellfish

Most shellfish allergies are lifelong with the onset occurring in adulthood. It's estimated that approximately 7 million people are allergic to shellfish. Shellfish are categorized as either crustaceans or mollusks. Crustaceans include shrimp, prawn, crayfish, crab, and lobster. Mollusks include clams, mussels, oysters, squid (calamari), cuttlefish, abalone, octopus, snails, sea urchin, and scallops.

In most cases, people are only allergic to one type of shellfish. For example, you might not be able to eat shrimp, yet you can eat octopus. However, for people with an allergy to any shellfish, it's recommended to avoid the entire category. It's important to work with your allergist to determine what's safe for you.

Fish with fins don't come from the same family as shellfish, so a person with a shellfish allergy isn't necessarily allergic to finned fish as well. Depending on the severity of your allergy, even touching shellfish or being near shellfish when it's cooked can cause a severe reactions like stomach cramping, vomiting, trouble breathing, hives, dizziness, confusion, or anaphylaxis.

Tree Nuts

Tree nuts include walnuts, almonds, cashews, pistachios, hazelnuts, macadamia, pine nuts, and Brazil nuts. Tree nuts differ from peanuts in that they grow on trees and not in the soil. Having an allergy to a specific tree nut increases your chances of being allergic to other types. It's recommended to avoid all nuts if you have a tree nut allergy, including peanuts, as there's a high chance of cross-contamination when these nuts are processed and manufactured. Nuts can be added to many different foods, so it's essential to read food labels carefully.

Allergic reactions can include abdominal pain, nausea, difficulty swallowing, itching of mouth, throat, eyes, or skin, as well as difficulty breathing. It can also lead to anaphylaxis.

FOODIE FACTOID

The FDA deemed the coconut should be labeled as a tree nut in 2006. Botanically a coconut is a "drupe," which is a fruit with a hard covering enclosing the seed. It's not botanically a nut, but is related to palm trees. There's disagreement between botanists and scientists as to the correct classification. However, some research suggests most people who are allergic to tree nuts can eat coconut. As with any food, be sure to check with your allergist or physician before adding coconuts into your diet.

Peanuts

One of the most common food allergies is to peanuts. This type of allergy is increasing in young children—between 1997 and 2008, peanut allergies in children more than tripled. The reaction to peanuts can be very severe and potentially fatal. Even the smallest amount of peanuts can cause a reaction. Contact with peanuts, such as touching a nut, is less likely to cause an extreme reaction. However, if the peanut residue comes in contact with the nose, mouth, or eyes, it's more of a concern and can possibly produce a more severe reaction.

Many people with peanut allergies carry EpiPens with them at all times and are required to strictly avoid all products containing peanuts. With any allergy, it's always important to read the ingredient list on food labels to ensure a product doesn't contain that specific ingredient. Peanut allergies generally have shown to be lifelong allergies. However, 20 percent of children with a peanut allergy have outgrown it.

Peanuts should not be confused with tree nuts. Peanuts grow underground and belong to the legume family, which includes peas, lentils, soybeans, and beans. Studies show that if you have a peanut allergy, you're more likely to also be allergic to tree nuts. However, if you have a peanut allergy, it doesn't necessarily mean you're allergic to other legumes such as beans and soy. The main reason some people with peanut allergies are also allergic to tree nuts is mostly due to cross-contamination during processing.

Because of the FDA's FALCPA law mentioned earlier, manufacturers must list if a food contains peanuts. However, anyone with allergies should continue to read all labels on all packages carefully. When in doubt, don't eat it. Symptoms can include a tingling sensation in the mouth or throat, nausea, congestion, rash, hives, or even anaphylaxis.

Eggs

Egg allergies are the second most common allergy seen in children. The American College of Allergy, Asthma, and Immunology estimates that 2 percent of children are allergic to eggs but many will outgrow it by age 16. It's actually the white of the egg that contains the proteins to which the body is reactive, but it's recommended to avoid eggs entirely if you have this allergy.

People with egg allergies should avoid eggs from ducks, geese, quails, and turkeys, in addition to chicken eggs. Reactions from an egg allergy occur after eating eggs or foods that contain eggs, and they occur within a few minutes to a few hours. Symptoms can include hives, nasal congestion, skin rashes, vomiting, digestive issues, and in very rare cases, anaphylactic shock.

Food products that can contain eggs:

Albumin	Lecithin
Baked goods	Marshmallows
Dried or powdered eggs	Mayonnaise
Eggnog	Meringue or meringue powder
Fresh pasta	

Soy

Soybeans belong to the legume family and include plants that have seeds or pods. A soybean allergy is considered one of the more common food allergies, and is seen in greater amounts in infants and children. Food Allergy Research and Education suggests that approximately 0.4 percent of children are allergic to soy, with most outgrowing it by the age of 10.

If you have a soy allergy, you're not necessarily allergic to other legumes. However, soybeans are used in a variety of processed food products, so it's important to thoroughly read food labels. Symptoms of an allergic reaction to soy can include tingling of the mouth, hives, itchy skin rash, wheezing, difficulty breathing, diarrhea, vomiting, nausea, abdominal pain, and/or swelling in the lips, mouth, or throat.

Foods that may contain soy include:

Baby formula	Soy milk
Baked goods	Soy sauce
Edamame	Tamari
Miso	Tempeh
Natto	Textured vegetable protein
Nutritional supplements	Tofu
Salad dressings	

The list of hidden soy can be very long, so checking an item's ingredients is essential.

Fortifying Your Diet

When you suffer from any type of food allergy, intolerance, or sensitivity and must leave out certain foods or food groups from your daily diet, it's important to fortify your diet with the nutrients you're missing from those foods. This is why working with a dietitian is essential when you have these issues. Not only can a dietitian help you avoid the foods you need to avoid, but he or she can help you replace them with foods that will continue to keep your diet healthy and well balanced.

Dairy Alternatives

Replacing dairy products is fairly easy due to the huge variety of dairy-free alternatives available in the marketplace. When selecting a product, one of the most important factors besides taste is fortification. Remember the dairy group contains vital nutrients like calcium and vitamin D. If you're unable to consume milk-based products, you need to get those nutrients elsewhere. Ensure the products you choose contain and/or are fortified with calcium and vitamin D.

Dairy-free alternatives can include:

Almond cheese	Honey butter
Almond milk	Nondairy, trans fat-free margarines
Coconut milk	Rice milk
Coconut oil	Soy milk
Grain-based milk	Vegan cheese

Egg Substitutes

Omitting eggs from your diet may seem pretty easy, especially if you think of eggs as a breakfast food. However, eggs are a common leavening agent, binder, and emulsifier, and are used in a staggering amount of recipes and food products available. Americans typically don't need to replace protein from eggs, as we tend to get sufficient protein from other sources as well as vitamin B_{12} and magnesium.

Egg binder replacement alternatives in baked goods include:

Agar

Arrowroot

Baking soda

Buttermilk

Commercial egg replacement
  powder

Ground flaxseeds

Mixtures of flour and oatmeal

Puréed fruits, such as bananas or
  applesauce

Soy lecithin

Tofu

Yogurt

Gluten-Free Foods

There are so many gluten-free products available on the market now, in addition to foods that are naturally gluten-free. Products such as breads, pastas, and baked goods can be close in texture and taste to their wheat-containing counterpart. Going gluten-free no longer has to be a food death sentence! But if you have celiac disease or a gluten intolerance, it's essential that you learn to read food labels and ingredient lists because there are thousands of gluten-containing ingredients, even if they're not labeled as gluten.

Gluten-free foods and ingredients include:

Amaranth

Arrowroot

Brown or white rice

Buckwheat flour

Chia flour

Chickpea flour

Coconut flour

Corn flour

Cornmeal

Hemp flour

Lupin flour

Maize flour

Millet flour

Oat flour—certified GF

Potato flour

Potato starch flour

Quinoa flour

Sorghum flour

Soya flour

Tapioca flour

Teff

FOODIE FACTOID

In 2013, the FDA issued a regulation that now defines the term "gluten-free" for food labeling, making gluten-free claims consistent and reliable across the food industry. Whether a food is manufactured to be gluten-free or it's naturally gluten-free, it can use the gluten-free labeling claim as long as it meets all FDA requirements resulting in less than 20 parts per million of gluten per serving for a gluten-free food.

Dining Out with a Food Allergy

Dining out should be an enjoyable experience. However, when a family member or friend has a serious food allergy, dining out has the potential to become a very dangerous experience. Today's restaurant guest with food allergies has more options for dining out. Most large chain restaurants provide allergen training for their staff, which makes them better able to accommodate patrons with food allergies. This training can include staff at the corporate office, as well as those who have determined what allergens are present in all of the supplier ingredients and have worked with the chefs to know if recipes and procedures need to be changed.

Smaller facilities may not have as strong training protocols in place and there may be much variability. Many restaurants post their menus and ingredient lists online. Other facilities may note on the menu which items can be substituted in place of an allergen. Finally, there are many food allergy support groups and websites that provide a list of suggestions for dining out.

NOTABLE INSIGHT

Go online to check out the following food allergy resources:

- foodallergy.org
- foodallergy.org/support-groups
- allergyeats.com
- cdc.gov/healthyyouth/foodallergies
- foodallergyednetwork.org
- aafa.org/esg_search.cfm

The Restaurant Selection Process

Choosing where to eat is always the first question when dining out. Ask friends who have food allergies where they've had a good dining experience. You need to take charge when venturing out to a new restaurant when you have an allergy. Never be afraid to ask your server questions before ordering or to order foods prepared in certain ways. Keep in mind that cross-contamination can always be an issue, so don't hesitate to ask how certain foods are cooked or what they're cooked in. Never assume!

It's a Team Effort

It takes a team effort to help create an allergy-friendly meal at a restaurant. From the restaurant being proactive and providing adequate allergy training for staff, to your careful restaurant selection, to you clearly communicating your health needs, it all leads to an enjoyable and safe food experience. You should always feel comfortable with the restaurant's staff and know that they're able to understand and meet your health needs. If not, don't eat there! Also, don't put yourself knowingly at risk if you have severe food allergies.

The Least You Need to Know

- Food allergies, food intolerances, and food sensitivities are all different.
- If you have a food affliction, you should work with a registered dietitian or nutritionist to learn what foods to avoid while still consuming a healthy and well-balanced diet.
- Many foods have hidden ingredients, so never assume that a food doesn't contain an allergen or a food to which you are sensitive or intolerant. Learn as much as you can concerning the foods you have problems with, so you know how to avoid them in all cases.
- Food allergies, sensitivities, and intolerances do not need to ruin your social life. With some determination and research, you can be prepared and still enjoy eating out.

Let's Get Cooking

Do you always find at the end of a long day you have no idea about what to make for dinner? You're not alone. It would be nice if your personal chef had a beautifully prepared and healthy meal on your table when you arrived home. But if the likelihood of having your own personal chef is slim to none, then you're going to have to make do by yourself.

In this chapter, we'll show you what you need to get a nutritious meal on the table in 30 minutes or less, simply by using a little organization and planning. We also give you some tips for keeping your kitchen organized and well supplied.

In This Chapter

- Where will your next meal come from?
- Stocking up for quick meals
- How to prep food efficiently and with ease
- Which cooking method is fastest?

Meal Planning Made Easy

Today it seems that everyone is short on time and many lack direction when it comes to planning healthy meals. As with any new project, you must start at the beginning. You need to be gentle with yourself, and know your limitations and capabilities. You also need to establish realistic goals or you'll be setting yourself up for failure. Meal planning actually can be made simple—you only need a plan of action.

Think Seasonally

The first step in meal planning is to think what healthy foods are in season. What fresh foods are being harvested now? What have you seen in the sale ads, in stores, or at the local farmer's market? By shopping seasonally, you'll save money and the produce will be at its peak of flavor.

It's helpful to get a seasonal produce calendar and keep it nearby for meal planning. Many produce calendars that are specific to your region can be found online. The following list provides a few top contenders for each season:

> **Spring:** Asparagus, broccoli, lettuce, peas, onions, and turnips
>
> **Summer:** Peppers, strawberries, summer squash, tomatoes, and eggplant
>
> **Fall:** Winter squash, chard, brussels sprouts, cranberries, and beets
>
> **Winter:** Oranges, kale, cabbage, parsnips, bok choy, and cauliflower

Finding the Time to Cook

To eat healthier, you must find the time to cook. Begin by evaluating your weekly schedule. Are there days that are more generally demanding than others? Do you have a meeting or activity that typically runs late? Which days do you have more time to devote to being in the kitchen? Answering these questions will help you budget your time and decide when you need to have ready-prepared foods on hand to create a nutritious meal in minutes.

Meal Solutions

In some cases, your schedule may be so overbooked that you need to call in a support team. You may need to recruit family members and assign them a day or a meal to cook. There are also options available for meal delivery services, which are shipped right to your door with all the ingredients to make a complete meal. Cooking classes also are available in some areas and you can make a week's worth of meals to take home to cook (or reheat and serve). If you're looking for a solution that takes even less time, there are companies in some cities where you can choose from a variety of nutrient-controlled breakfasts, lunches, dinners, and snacks you can take home and reheat.

Grocery stores are even trying to help consumers eat better, too. You can purchase a variety of fresh fruits and vegetables washed, sliced, diced, and ready to use. Many stores have elaborate ready-to-eat food counters with everything from fresh salads to home-style soups. Their consumer-friendly vegetables can be real timesavers in the kitchen.

 FOODIE FACTOID

In 1940, Irving Naxon invented what we now refer to as the Crock-pot, or slow cooker. It was originally called the Naxon Beanery. This kitchen appliance is very popular with those who don't like to spend a lot of time over a hot stove.

Kitchen Organization

One way to gobble up your time is to cook in a poorly organized kitchen. If you have trouble finding a square inch of usable work surface in your kitchen, you need to spend a couple of hours getting organized. Ideally you should remove anything that doesn't belong in the kitchen. Next evaluate the equipment on the counters, peek in your utensil drawer, and review your pot and pan storage. Is what you use most often where you can easily access it? If not, reorganize it so the most used items are located front and center.

A Well-Stocked Pantry

At least once or twice annually, you should sort through your pantry, whether it be a cabinet or a few shelves. Organize your items into stations, such as canned goods, baking supplies, spices and condiments, pasta and rice, snack foods, breakfast foods, and so on. It's also a good idea to invest in either plastic or metal shelf risers to allow you to double your space and be able to actually view your supplies. The following table provides a great start to a well-stocked pantry.

Basic Food Pantry

Canned Goods	Dry Goods	Flavorings
Black beans	Brown rice	Salt
Pinto beans	Jasmine rice	Pepper
Garbanzo beans	Spaghetti	Italian seasonings
Green beans	Angel hair pasta	Curry powder
Green peas	Macaroni noodles	Cinnamon
Corn	Couscous	Coriander
Diced tomatoes	Quinoa	Cumin
Whole tomatoes	Oats	Red pepper flakes
Tomato sauce	All-purpose flour	Chili powder
Tomato paste	Whole wheat flour	Soy sauce
Chicken stock	Brown sugar	Ponzu
Vegetable stock	Sugar	Mustard
Roasted peppers	Baking powder	Mayonnaise
Soups	Baking soda	Ketchup
	Chocolate chips	Salsa
	Shredded coconut	Olive oil
	Tofu (shelf-stable)	Canola oil

Additional items, such as onions, garlic, and potatoes, should be kept in a cool, dark place like a pantry. Keep these items in a separate bin for easy cleanup.

From this basic pantry list, you should be able to put a meal on the table in 30 minutes or less. Additionally, you need to keep your refrigerator and freezer stocked with the following basics:

Cold Storage: Butter, shredded cheese, eggs, milk or milk alternatives, lemons, limes, and oranges.

Freezer Storage: Lean proteins such as flash-frozen chicken breasts or fish fillets, and ground meats such as turkey, chicken, beef, and pork.

Creating Your Meal Plan

If meal planning is new to you, you're going to want to ease into it. Start with a goal of planning meals for two or three days per week. Ideally you'll cook twice and plan to have sufficient ingredients to create the Day 3 quick-assembly meal that requires no cooking or just a simple reheat.

Follow these 10 steps to planning your meals:

1. Decide which days you want to have meals for and write them down on a notepad or dry erase board in your kitchen.

2. On your list, separate each day into breakfast, lunch, dinner, and two snacks.

3. Decide on a protein source for each main meal and write it down.

4. Look at your seasonal produce guide and select fruit and vegetables for each main meal.

5. Research recipes online to get ideas for your key recipe ingredients and print out the ones you need. Also look at the sale ads or what's available at your local farmers market.

6. Determine what foods you can cook extra amounts of that you can repurpose for the next mealtime. For example, if you grill chicken on Sunday, can you grill an extra piece to add to your vegetable salad at lunch the next day?

7. Review the meal plan and recipes to ensure it makes sense for your week time-wise and for your skill level.

8. Round out your meals with additional whole grains, fruits, and vegetables to create a well-balanced meal. Make sure each meal is colorful.

9. Create your shopping list. Write down all the ingredients required in your recipes, then verify what you have in stock.

10. Go shopping, and when you return home put everything away promptly.

Meal planning will take some getting acquainted with, so be sure to allow yourself a little extra time to get into a routine. If you try to do too much too fast, it could be a bit overwhelming and you might get discouraged.

Food Prep Made Easy

Now that your kitchen is well organized, it will be a joy to get to work. As you review your meal plan, think about your meals and recipes and ask yourself if there are certain tasks you can prepare ahead that will save you time later when you're cooking meal. For many people, it's the chopping of produce that's daunting. You can do up to a week's worth at a time of durable veggies and store it in the fridge. You can also use a food processor or purchase vegetables prewashed and prechopped. Another great timesaver is to always cook and freeze extra rice or whole grains to pull out for use in another meal.

What's the Best Way to Cook?

Depending on your recipe, there's more than one way to cook your dishes. Which method you use depends on your personal style and how much time you have. Just about every method can be an everyday healthy way to cook, with only one exception—frying.

Sautéing

French for "jump in the pan," this quick-cooking method is great for getting the meal on the table fast. To use this method, add a little oil to the pan, and heat until it begins to shimmer. When the oil is hot enough, you'll hear a sizzle when you add the food to the pan. Sautéing is a great method for cooking just about anything that's tender and needs a short amount of cooking time, such as vegetables and thin pieces of meat or fish.

Grilling

Outdoor cooking and barbecuing has always been popular, but it's also a great way to add additional layers of flavor to foods. While it does require a little bit of setup, the payoff is worth it. The most important step is to first oil down the grill grates with vegetable oil to help prevent your food from sticking. Next, heat your grill to medium high heat. Lean meat like chicken is a great choice for the grill. Pat the chicken dry and lay it out on a sheet pan. Season it and place the sheet pan on the grill with the lid off and cook the chicken to an internal temperature of 165°F. It's imperative to use a digital meat thermometer to end up with moist and juicy chicken that's thoroughly cooked. In the last 10 minutes of cooking, brush on your favorite sauce.

Vegetables are also delicious when grilled. The key to grilling vegetables is to ensure the pieces are large enough to turn over with the tongs and that they aren't so small they fall through the grate.

 FOODIE FACTOID

The safe minimum food temperatures for protein foods are:

- Chicken breast: 165°F
- Hamburger: 160°F
- Beef steak: 145°F
- Fish: 145°F
- Pork: 145°F

Steaming

There are many ways to steam foods in your kitchen. You can steam on the stovetop in a pan filled with a little water and a metal or silicone steamer insert; in a bamboo steamer over a pot; in a microwave steamer tray; or in an electric steamer that can cook multiple layers of foods. Whichever one you own is a great way to cook food fast and retain nutrients. Steam is hotter than air, so it takes less time to cook, too.

Using a microwave steamer at work is a great way to cook a hot meal fast. Because it adds moisture to the food, meat proteins don't get as tough during the cooking process. Be sure to microwave your foods to 165°F for food safety.

Baking

Baking is a dry-heat cooking method. Heat is transferred from the outside of the food to the inside. Convection baking incorporates a fan to circulate the air evenly around the food, so it provides excellent browning and cooks it faster. When converting recipes between the two types, reduce the temperature of a convection oven by 25°F since it cooks faster. Because cooking time is less, be sure to keep a close eye on your recipe. Baking is a great all-purpose way to cook everything from chicken and fish to casseroles and muffins.

Frying

Frying is also a dry-heat method because the food is submerged in hot oil. It works by heating the liquid in the food into steam. When fried foods are cooked at the proper temperature, they don't absorb much fat. However, improperly cooked foods will act as a sponge and absorb excess oil. It's important to maintain the correct frying temperature to prevent prolonged cooking in the oil. The general frying temperature is about 350°F. This is not the healthiest cooking method to use, but it does make foods crispy.

Sous Vide

Sous vide (under vacuum) is one of the newest and coolest cooking techniques. Vacuum-sealed food is cooked in a temperature-controlled water bath over many hours at a low temperature. It produces perfectly cooked moist and tender food. However, this method isn't for everyone, as it takes a long time to cook and the units can cost upwards of $400.

Order's Up

Now that you've spent the day preparing and cooking foods for the week, what are you going to do with it all? It's time to get it packaged up for easy eating. Gather all of your supplies such as your measuring cups, scale, containers, labels, and a marker, and get ready for the week. One thing to consider is how you're going to reheat the food. You also need to look at the order in which you intend to eat your week's worth of prepared foods. Plan to eat the more delicate items or those that begin to lose their texture the first few days and save the more durable items like stews for later.

A large piece of chicken breast is going to dry out before it gets evenly heated throughout. The solution would be to preslice it before putting it into your microwave-safe container. It would also be helpful to add other ingredients (side dishes) with a little moisture. Try to keep everything about the same size piece-wise so the foods will reheat evenly.

Some recipes don't require any cook time and are ready to eat. However, think about if you make a fruit parfait with yogurt—you're going to need different containers to prevent the granola from getting soggy. The same is true for salads—keep the dressing on the side and mix it right before eating. A little bit of thought and planning on the front end will make eating a joy.

Portion Sizes

As you compose your balanced meals of vegetables, fruits, whole grains, and lean proteins, make sure to weigh out foods on your scale or use your measuring cups to get just the right size portion. Allow yourself a little extra time for this step. After you've practiced packaging your meals a few times, you'll be able to identify correct portions on sight.

Leftovers

How long should you keep leftovers? Well, it depends on the food. Most prepped or prepared foods can be kept for 7 days in the refrigerator. Now that doesn't mean it will be at its peak flavor or texture at Day 7, it simply means it won't make you ill.

If you pack your lunch, use freezer packs in your lunch tote to keep it cool. Food should never be left out for more than 2 hours in the danger zone between 40° and 140°F. If you end up not eating your packed lunch that day and it remained unrefrigerated in your lunch tote, you need to toss it out. Be food safe and don't risk getting sick over it.

The Least You Need to Know

- Meal planning should be fun. Don't be afraid to seek out help when it comes to meal preparation. It's a great way to involve the family.
- A organized and well-stocked kitchen with the right tools makes cooking a lot more fun and saves time.
- Choose the best way to healthily cook your meals.

Eating Out

Dining out can have many pitfalls when you're following a healthy diet. Selecting the perfect restaurant can be a balance between what you're craving and what you know you should select. It's important to be prepared and conscious of how the experience appeals to your senses and emotions.

A few simple rules will help you be successful with a healthy diet when you dine out. Pass on the breadbasket or bottomless chips. Sip on your water and enjoy the atmosphere and company. When the food comes, eat slowly and savor the experience. Dining out isn't just about the food. It's about the environment, enjoying being waited on, and socializing.

In This Chapter

- How to eat out with healthfulness in mind
- Navigating restaurant menus
- Avoiding overindulgence at the bar
- Identifying the best on-the-go food choices

Frequency of Meals Away from Home

According to the U.S. Department of Agriculture (USDA), eating one meal a week away from home contributes an additional 134 calories a week to your diet or about 2 pounds per year. That's 10 pounds every 5 years. In addition to the additional calories, dining out increases your sodium, saturated fat, added sugar, and alcohol intake. On average, foods eaten away from home contribute to an overall decrease in the quality of the diet, including a decreased consumption of fruit, some vegetable groups, and whole grains by an average of 25 percent.

Whether you contribute to the increase or not, eating out is a social event and cultural phenomenon. Look back over the last month and ask yourself how many times you ate away from home at a restaurant. On the surface, it may seem you don't eat out often, but when you start breaking it down to a morning latte a couple of times a week, lunch with co-workers twice a week, happy hour on Friday, brunch on Sunday, and a frequent takeout pizza night, it starts to add up.

Eating out on a regular basis and still maintaining a healthy diet can be difficult. Eating the majority of your meals and calories at home will be easier on your waistline and your wallet. Save dining out for special occasions and social events. If you think of eating out as "dining out," the event becomes more meaningful.

If you regularly grab a meal on the run, it defintely will take time to curtail those urges and habits. Making good new habits will help change old ones. Instead of going out to lunch at work, gather a group of co-workers to go on a walk during lunchtime. Plan an after-work hike instead of happy hour. Think of social activities not centered around food.

Reducing your frequency of eating out is the goal; however, when the occasion arises you will still need to have tools to help make your dining experience healthy. Planning ahead can help you be successful. Choose your restaurant wisely, look at the menu before you arrive, and eat something small 1 to 2 hours before leaving so you won't be starving when you are seated.

Selecting a Restaurant

Dining out can seem like you're running through a field of landmines. Being unprepared can lead to consumption of high calories, fat, and sodium. With a little preparation ahead of time, you can eat out occasionally and not sabotage your diet.

Choosing the restaurant is the first step. Your goal is to find a place with a good selection of healthy options in normal-sized portions. Sounds easy enough, right? Depends on what restaurants are on your area. You will likely have to expand your horizons and try out some new places. However, dining out at a new place can actually help you order healthier.

Use apps listing local restaurants in your area. You can search using a keyword such as "healthy" to find options near you. Such apps will show reviews and pictures of the restaurant's food along customer ratings. You may even be able to view their menu and possibly even the nutritional information.

FOODIE FACTOID

The National Restaurant Association reports an increase in the use of smartphones and tablets by its consumers. Of those individuals owning this technology, 14% of millennials and 19% of baby boomers look up nutrition information on an app at least once a week. Many of these users are also receiving special deals and coupons and paying for their meals through the app.

Looking for the obvious healthier restaurants may make your ordering decision easier. Fish and seafood restaurants will have a large selection of fish and generally offer a wide variety of cooking methods to enhance the food's flavor without heavy sauces.

Places with large salad bars can be a healthy diner's paradise, but watch out for pitfalls. Bacon, cheese, croutons, olives, and heavy dressings can add fat, calories, and sodium to an otherwise healthy salad. Use caution when building your salad. Choose oil and vinegar in bottles for your salads in place of dressings. Don't pour the dressing directly on your salad; instead, look for small cups to fill and use the "dip your fork" method when eating. If the salad is also your meal, add protein to it. If chicken isn't available, choose to add beans and hard-boiled eggs.

Many restaurants are cognizant that consumers want healthier options and include healthy foods on their menu. You don't have to limit yourself to dining only at health-focused restaurants. Learning how to order, using restraint, and making good choices will allow you to eat healthy at almost any restaurant.

Both small and large chain restaurants are appealing to health-focused consumers by listing nutritional information on their websites. Be prepared by looking at options *before* you arrive at the restaurant. Use caution when you look at nutritional information online. Read the description carefully and take note if condiments, salad dressings, and sides are included in the information. These may be listed separately, so you will need to add these to the final calorie count.

The Food Dialogue

The wait staff is the liaison between you and the kitchen. Don't be shy about asking your server for help. Let your server know immediately that you're looking for healthy options. Many will be well versed on options they can provide and help you with your selection. If they can't answer questions, ask them (very nicely) to find out from the kitchen. Often the kitchen is happy to accommodate with a varied method of cooking, sauces on the side, and not salting vegetables. Even with recommendations from your server, continue to use your own judgment.

A Quick Guide to Meal Selection

Looking at menus online before you get to the restaurant will speed up the selection process. If menus are not available or you're eating out on the spur of the moment, there are some tricks you can use to quickly select the healthiest option on the menu.

Look for the "light" section of the menu. Not all restaurants will have one, and sometimes the foods will be denoted with a symbol and mixed into their traditional subcategories. Finding these items on the menu, if available, at least guarantees the item you choose will be lighter than their average entrée. Many lighter menu selections are generally around 600 calories or less. Icons may depict a variety of health-conscious choices, which may include include healthy, low-sodium, vegetarian, or heart-healthy options.

The American Heart Association has a heart checkmark icon that restaurants can use to note if a menu selection meets certain nutritional standards. This red heart with a white checkmark inside indicates the menu items meet the AMA's standards on calories, fat, saturated fat, trans fat, and sodium, and contain a beneficial nutrient.

Words to Watch For

Descriptive words are used to paint a picture in the diner's mind and tantalize the taste buds. These words can help lead you down the path to healthy choices. Not every menu item using these words will be a healthy option (baked mac-n-cheese, for example). Use them as a guide to look for healthier items:

- 100% whole wheat
- Baked
- Blackened
- Broiled
- Grilled
- Light
- Marinara
- Poached

- Red sauce
- Roasted
- Seared
- Seasoned (could have added salt)
- Steamed
- Stir-fried (ask for sauces on the side)
- Vinaigrette
- Whole wheat or whole grain

Avoiding fried foods is an easy way to make your choices healthier. However, it isn't always easy to tell from the description. The following is a list of words to help uncover which foods are or may be fried:

- Battered
- Breaded
- Crispy
- Crunchy
- Deep-fried
- Pan-fried

Fat isn't always a bad thing, as we've discussed—there are beneficial fats. Dining out and choosing the wrong menu item can cause you to surpass your daily cap of saturated fat without thinking. Cheese is healthy in moderation, but a serving is a 1-inch cube. Not many restaurant dishes containing cheese limit it to one serving. Added butter will also wreak havoc on your max of fat for the day. Check out the following list for keywords to clue you in to added fat from cream, cheese, and butter:

- à la mode (served with ice cream)
- au fromage (with cheese)
- au gratin (topped with breadcrumbs, cheese, butter, and eggs)
- au lait (prepared or served with milk)
- Basted
- Béarnaise
- Buttery or buttered
- Cheese sauce
- Creamy
- Creamy or creamed
- Gooey
- Hollandaise
- Loaded
- Melted
- Newburg
- Rich
- Sautéed
- Scalloped
- Smothered
- Stuffed
- Thermidor
- Velvety
- White sauce

Added sugar can be just as detrimental to a healthy diet as added fat. Watch out for sweet sauces, toppers, and added sugar with the following words:

- BBQ
- Glazed
- Honey
- Honey mustard
- Maple

- Sticky
- Sweet and sour
- Sweetened
- Teriyaki

Avoid portion distortion by skipping items including the phrases all you can eat, bottomless, giant, and super size.

Words that sound too good to be true may be just that. You should use caution when you see descriptions including "free" (fat-free, sugar-free, carb-free) on a menu. In these meals, the calories come either from fat, carbohydrate, or protein. If one energy group is lacking, it's made up for in the other groups.

WAKE-UP CALL

According to PBS, the low-fat craze hit America in the 1990s following reports that Americans were ingesting too much fat. There was not a differentiation between heart-healthy fats, trans fats, and saturated fats at that time. Consumers responded by switching to low-fat and fat-free items, believing these were better for them. Consumers falsely believed that as long as a food did not have fat, it was healthy. The problem with removing fat from items is it has to be replaced with another ingredient to make it palatable. This ingredient was often sugar or processed carbohydrate, neither of which is healthy in large quantities.

Navigating the Menu for Good Health

Learning how to choose a restaurant, watching out for unhealthy description words, and looking for healthy food symbols on a menu will help you enjoy the dining-out experience without sacrificing your new lifestyle. Now you need to learn how to navigate the menu.

Appetizers

The original role of the appetizer was to stimulate the appetite. Only a few small bites were eaten prior to the first course. Currently, appetizers now are generally very high in calories and fat, and if entire portions are eaten, they often quench your appetite rather than stimulate it.

If you must order an appetizer, choose wisely. Look for items made with vegetables close to their natural state. Select ones with healthy fats, high nutrient content, and good sources of lean protein.

Entrées

Portion distortion is one of the biggest problems you may be faced with when you eat out. The gigantic plates are filled with enough food for at least two meals. Consider sharing an entrée with your dining companion, or ask for a to-go box right away and take home half your meal. If they're available, order half-size or lunch-size servings.

Look for the lighter entrées. Most dining establishments offer a "lighter" section on their menu. Read the small print and don't take this as permission to eat your entire entrée. Sometimes these entrées are still 600 calories. Share an entrée with your dining companion and ask wait staff to split it onto two plates.

Here are some guidelines for selecting the better options on menus. Entrées should be:

- 600 calories or less (you can still share or take part home)
- 6g of saturated fat or less
- 900mg of sodium or less

Be sure to read descriptions for items thoroughly, and ask for clarification on words you're unsure of. Request that items be brought without high-calorie options like sauces and toppings. You can also ask for items such as cheese, olives, and nuts on the side. Using these items in moderation is perfectly okay; however, entrées and salads generally have more than a serving of these items on them.

Not all calories are equal. Calories from avocado, cheese, and nuts are not the same as calories from bacon, dressing, and sauces. When you look at nutritional information, consider what is the source of calories in the dish. If your choice is a nutrient-packed food, then moderation is fine. A grilled salmon sandwich may seem high in calories and fat, but the fat is the healthy omega-3.

Sides

Sides can add calories, fat, and sodium very quickly to your otherwise healthy entrée. Most servers will happily substitute fresh fruit or a small side salad for fries or other unhealthy sides. Request double vegetables instead of rice or another starch on the side. Look for additional vegetable sides you can order.

Desserts

Getting out of the habit of ordering dessert every time you go out is the best rule. Reserve dessert for special occasions. Many restaurants offer mini portions of famous desserts served in shot-size glasses. This is a great alternative to ordering a giant piece of cake. Pass a couple around to your table and have a bite of two or three different ones.

If you can't get past the craving, look for healthier options. Other options are available and may not be listed on the dessert menu. Look for:

- Fresh fruit plate with cheese
- A small scoop of sorbet, gelato, sherbet, or ice cream
- Poached fruit or baked apples
- Fruit tarts and pies (skip the crust and ice cream on the side)
- Coffee or cappuccino

The bottom line is the serving size. A couple of bites are not going to derail your success.

Cocktails

Ordering cocktails is a slippery slope when you're trying to maintain a healthy diet. You have options when you're faced with the inevitable social situation. If your companions are drinking and you feel the need to join them, consider ordering a nonalcoholic beverage such as seltzer with lime.

If you choose to order alcohol, think about the drink before you order. There are some beverages with fewer calories than others. Look for light versions of cocktails, such as skinny margaritas. You may also consider ordering a drink you would only sip slowly, such as a martini or a glass of red wine. Light beers are also lower in calories and fill you up more than a martini.

 FOODIE FACTOID

Here's an easy way to precisely determine the number of calories in your drink: the proof of alcohol multiplied by 0.8 multiplied by the number of ounces in a drink.

For example, if you have 1.5 ounces of 80 proof vodka:

$80 \times .8 \times 1.5 = 96$ calories

Don't forget to add the number of calories in your mixer.

If you consume alcoholic beverages, always do so in moderation (no more than one per day for women and two per day for men). At the end of the day, having one of your favorite cocktails or beers occasionally won't derail your healthy lifestyle.

Food on the Go

As Americans, we're constantly eating on the go—it's part of our culture. Learning to be mindful throughout our day is crucial to a healthy lifestyle. Being mindful when eating on the road can be very difficult.

Do you stop every morning at your favorite coffee shop for your morning latte? A large latte with whole milk and flavored syrup can run upwards of 500 calories. If eliminating it isn't an option, you'll need to rethink your drink. Start by ordering one size smaller. Next, switch out the milk. By moving down to 1% milk, you'll save calories and saturated fat. Consider reducing the amount of syrup in your drink or switch to sugar-free.

Smoothies are a fine meal substitute, but be cautious of calories. Try light versions without added sherbet. Often smoothies satisfy you for a few hours, but not as much as a meal would.

Fast food isn't always the best option, but it can be unavoidable. Here are some guidelines:

- Order a small hamburger
- Have a grilled chicken sandwich
- Skip the mayonnaise and use mustard instead
- Order a sandwich with lettuce and tomatoes
- Eat a side salad instead of fries
- Order chili without cheese

Submarine sandwiches can be a great option for eating on the go. Choose lean meats such as turkey and grilled chicken. Load up on vegetables and choose your condiments wisely. Mustard and vinegar (without the oil) are better choices than mayonnaise and dressings. Choose cheese in moderation. Order 100 percent whole wheat bread if it's offered and consider removing the top half of the bun.

Breakfast on the go also has some great options. Many fast-food outlets and coffee shops offer oatmeal, yogurt parfaits, and healthy breakfast wraps or sandwiches. Look for yogurt parfaits made with Greek yogurt and nuts as the topping. When choosing breakfast sandwiches, there's no need to forgo the whole egg and order only egg whites. However, often egg-white wraps or sandwiches are offered in conjunction with healthier options such as a whole-grain muffin. Skip the fatty breakfast meats. A slice of cheese is a better option than ham or bacon.

Meals at the Grocery Store

Shopping at the grocery store isn't just for raw foods anymore. The grocery store is packed full of ready-to-eat items. Grocery store chains have gone out of their way to appeal to the harried consumer wanting to grab a meal and go.

The deli section is an obvious first place to start. Fruit salad, tomato caprese, roasted vegetables, and tabbouleh salad are all available by the pound. Many full-service deli counters offer pre cooked salmon, grilled chicken breasts, and whole roasted chickens. These are generally higher in sodium than you would make at home, but they're great alternatives to takeout or restaurant foods.

Frozen foods are another option. Read labels to determine what fits your lifestyle and diet. There are a wide variety of options available. Look for light versions of frozen pizza, precooked chicken, and vegetables without sauces.

If you want to do a little more of the cooking yourself but want foods already prepped, shop around the outer aisles of the store for great options. The produce section has prepackaged salads, precut vegetables and fruit, and ready-to-roast vegetable mixes. The butcher's counter has premade kabobs and premarinated chicken breasts ready to throw on the grill.

The Least You Need to Know

- Dining out can be a wonderful experience if you plan ahead and research sensible choices.
- Good communication skills can help restaurant servers understand your dietary needs.
- Ordering from the appetizer and sides sections of the menu can mean smaller portion sizes, which typically equal fewer calories.
- Meals on the go can be healthier if you take the time to seek out better options.
- Check out the healthy food selections offered at your neighborhood grocery store for ready-to-eat meals and snacks.

What Science Says About Special Foods

Are there any good diets out there? In this part, we explore the most popular diets and look at their strengths and weaknesses, along with their impact on health. You'll also learn how foods obtain "superfood" status, and we'll examine the specific nutrients that make them super.

In this part, we'll also take a look into common farm and ranch practices for growing and raising foods, and the ways animals are handled. We'll investigate the use of antibiotics and growth hormones, along with policies and regulations that control them. Additionally, you'll learn about sustainable food practices, aquaculture, and various systems' environmental impacts.

Alcohol and coffee are always in the news and in everyone's hands. Are they beneficial to health or harmful? A review of the risks and benefits of this type of controversial foods will be explored. Additionally, we'll discuss the consumption of alcohol in healthy individuals, and also the risk it poses for heart disease and breast cancer.

Top Diets

With the beginning of each year it seems that a brand-new diet plan is released. Should you follow it or not? Who's promoting it and why? Is it easy to use and is it a safe and nutritious way to lose weight? It's important to know the answers before starting a diet.

In this chapter, we'll discuss popular diets routinely reported about in books, magazines, and on television and the internet. You'll learn the basic components of the diets and how they define themselves. We'll also cover how easy they are to maintain and what costs you'll incur by following them.

In This Chapter

- A review of the science behind plant-based diets
- What ancient cavemen diets revealed
- Vegetarian diets and nutritional concerns
- A look at low-carbohydrate diets
- How commercial weight loss plans work

Plant-Based Diets

Plant-based diets are all the buzz in the nutrition world. They're popular with environmentalists, animal rights supporters, *locavores,* and dietitians. There are various degrees of plant-based diets from raw vegan to Mediterranean.

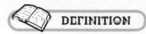 **DEFINITION**

> A **locavore** is a person who prefers to consume foods grown locally, generally within a 100-mile radius. Locavores support their local farmers by shopping at farmers markets and stores showcasing local ingredients. Living in an area with a mild climate makes being a locavore much easier than in areas with harsh winters.

A plant-based diet is exactly what it sounds like—the diet's primary (or exclusive) source of calories comes from plant products. Foods with very little processing are emphasized and items such as nuts, legumes, soy, whole grains, fruits, and vegetables are given the spotlight.

According to the Academy of Nutrition and Dietetics (AND), the term "vegetarianism" applies to plant-based diets as a whole. Over 47 percent of Americans report that they eat a vegetarian meal at least once a week. A study published in the *Journal of Family Medicine* reported that individuals with coronary heart disease who followed a plant-based diet as part of their therapy for a period of more than 3½ years saw a reduction in cardiac events.

The American Institute of Cancer Research recommends eating plant-based meals for at least two thirds of the calories you consume. By increasing your intake of fruits, vegetables, whole grains, and beans, you'll increase your fiber intake and fill up on foods that are not dense in calories. The institute also states that eating a mostly plant-based diet will not only help prevent cancer, but also will likely decrease your weight.

The Mediterranean Diet

The Mediterranean Diet is a lifelong way of eating. Based on the dietary patterns of countries bordering the Mediterranean Sea, this way of eating has been the subject of numerous studies. A multitude of research has concluded that following a Mediterranean diet will decrease the likelihood of death from cardiovascular disease and cancer. Additional research has shown a reduction in the incidence of Parkinson's and Alzheimer's diseases.

Following the patterns of a plant-based diet, each meal in the Mediterranean diet is based on fruits, vegetables, whole grains, legumes, nuts, and seeds. The following simple concepts are incorporated into the diet:

- Healthy fats, such as olive oil, replace butter and margarine.

- Foods are seasoned with herbs and spices instead of salt.

- Protein consists of frequent servings of fish and seafood at least twice a week.

- Additional proteins consumed include chicken, eggs, cheese, and yogurt.

- Dairy should be low fat or nonfat.

- Meat and sweets are eaten no more than a few times a month.

- Wine, typically red, is consumed in moderation. Moderation means no more than 5 ounces a day for women and men older than 65 (10 ounces a day for men under 65 years old).

Following this eating pattern is a way of life for many Mediterranean-based cultures. It's fairly easy to follow once you get accustomed to making choices that are in line with the diet. Most restaurants have options following these patterns, but you may need to ask for substitutions. Like most healthy ways of eating, you'll need to plan ahead and spend some time cooking. Learning simple trade-offs will become second nature. Try some of the following tips for a smooth transition:

- Replace mayonnaise with hummus.

- Add a handful of almonds to your yogurt.

- Incorporate legumes into meals.

- Try new salt-free seasoning blends.

- Dip your bread in small amounts of olive oil instead of margarine or butter.

People of the Mediterranean area are also active on a daily basis. They incorporate daily activities like riding a bike to the store or walking to the park into their lifestyle. Fitting physical activity into your daily life is a key component.

 FOODIE FACTOID

Hummus is synonymous with the Mediterranean diet. This ancient spread dates back as far as the twelfth or thirteenth century. The true country of origin is much debated—several Mediterranean countries claim bragging rights. However, the taste of hummus varies from region to region. It consists of chickpeas (garbanzo beans), sesame paste (tahini), lemon juice, salt, and garlic. Greeks use olive oil as an added fat, while Turks use butter. Some regions add Greek yogurt, chili peppers, or cumin. Hummus is a great addition to any diet, and passes the vegan test. Be careful to not overindulge in the tasty spread, it may be packed with nutrients, but it also is high in calories.

The Flexitarian Diet

The combination of a flexible diet and a vegetarian diet is called a flexitarian diet. Also referred to as "semi-vegetarian," a flexitarian follows a vegetarian diet in some form, but will occasionally eat meat. The subgroup of vegetarianism (*lacto-, ovo-, pesco-*) they follow on a daily basis, and how often they deviate from it, will determine the health benefits and what supplements they may need.

The flexitarian mind-set doesn't eliminate any foods or food groups, but rather adds more of the plant-based foods such as tofu, beans, nuts, and seeds. Being a plant-based diet, it focuses on fruits, vegetables, legumes, and grains.

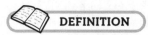 **DEFINITION**

> Words are added before "vegetarian" to clarify foods eaten outside of what a strict vegetarian would eat. **Lacto-vegetarians** adds dairy to their diet, **ovo-vegetarians** eat eggs, and **pesco-vegetarians** consume fish. Sometimes the prefixes are combined if an individual eats more than one category. For example, a lacto-ovo vegetarian eats a vegetarian diet but includes dairy and eggs.

The Vegetarian Diet

Strict vegetarians closely follow a more vegan diet. Plant-based foods such as grains, fruits, vegetables, and legumes comprise the majority of a vegetarian's calories.

According to AND, the bioavailability of plant-based protein should not be a concern for vegetarians or vegans. AND reports that protein from plant-based sources (such as beans, whole grains, nuts, and seeds) contains a sufficient supply of all the essential amino acids. Protein sources should include those recommended for vegans as well as any chosen by a particular subgroup, such as dairy, eggs, or fish.

Ensuring adequate intake of all minerals and vitamins is essential with any diet, and there are some considerations for vegetarians. Depending on the form of vegetarianism you follow, you may need to take supplements to ensure you're getting adequate vitamins and minerals.

Adequate amounts of omega-3 fatty acids can be ingested through nuts, seeds, avocado, flaxseeds, and healthy oils. For pesco-vegetarians, fish is an excellent source.

Iron is plentiful in animal products. With the elimination of these from the diet, iron deficiency becomes a cause for concern. Nonheme iron is the primary source of iron for vegetarians. Good sources include dark leafy vegetables, beans, and iron-fortified bread. Fiber and phytic acid, found in many fruits and vegetables, can inhibit the absorption of nonheme iron. Eating foods rich in vitamin C, such as citrus, tomatoes, and strawberries, will help with the absorption of iron. Zinc, also commonly found in animal-based products, may require supplementation.

There's also a high prevalence of vitamin B_{12} deficiency in both vegetarians and vegans. Deficiency symptoms include numbness and tingling in the hands and legs, fatigue, mood swings, an altered state of balance, irregular menstrual cycles, and memory difficulties. It's important to seek out top sources of B_{12}, however, supplementation may be necessary.

If dairy is eliminated from the vegetarian diet, there will likely be a decreased intake of calcium and vitamin D. Increasing consumption of dark-green vegetables (kale, spinach, and broccoli), beans, calcium-fortified juice, and milk substitute will ensure their calcium intake will be within dietary guidelines. Adequate vitamin D intake is difficult to achieve through diet. Sunlight is a valuable source, but supplementation may need to be considered.

 WAKE-UP CALL

Due to early research showing a possible link between omnivore diets and an increased risk of osteoporosis, there is some thought in the vegan community that their calcium needs may be lower than those for omnivores. The Vegetarian Resource Group states that vegans and vegetarians should follow the same calcium guidelines set by the U.S. Department of Agriculture (USDA) as meat eaters. Drinking calcium-fortified juice and soy milk as well as eating dark-green leafy vegetables will help with calcium intake, but a calcium supplement may still be needed.

Following a vegetarian diet has gotten easier over the years. School lunch programs, airlines, and restaurants all generally offer vegetarian selections. Carefully read menus and request alterations such as substituting black beans for chicken on a salad. To follow a healthy diet, you still must plan ahead and cook at home. Relying on meatless fast-food options can add unwanted calories, fat, and sodium to your diet. Because vegetarian diets are not as strict as a vegan diet, the cost shouldn't be any more than a traditional diet. In fact, the cost may even be less because you'll bypass the meat counter.

When following a vegetarian diet, remember that just because a food or meal is vegetarian doesn't mean it's healthy. Soda, candy, movie theater popcorn, and your vanilla soy latte are all vegetarian. Embrace the true vegetarian diet and eat a wide variety of nutrient-filled whole foods.

The Vegan Diet

Individuals choose a vegan diet for a variety of reasons. These may include social, animal rights, or environmental concerns, and/or health beliefs. Vegan individuals vary in degrees on how strictly they adhere to a true vegan diet. The basic premise is that no animal products of any kind, including butter, cheese, eggs, and honey (made by bees), are eaten. These include ingredients added to many products, such as whey, gelatin, and lard.

FOODIE FACTOID

Many acclaimed bakers around the world use butter as one of the basic ingredients for baking. If you are a baker and are going vegan, don't panic. There are butter alternatives on the market, or you can make your own. Keep in mind butter alternatives are still high in saturated fat and calories. They may also contain trans fats from hydrogenated oil.

Protein sources are strictly plant-based and include grains (quinoa, millet, and amaranth), legumes, tofu, soy, nuts and nut butters, and seeds. Due to eliminating all animal-based proteins, vegans should ensure they have adequate iron and zinc intake.

As noted with vegetarians, vegans may be at risk for developing several additional nutrient deficiencies. The addition of foods to compensate for the elimination of other groups is essential to maintaining good nutrition. Consider your sources and intake of calcium, iron, B_{12}, and zinc.

The degree to which you follow a true vegan diet and your support from friends and family will define the ease and longevity of following a vegan lifestyle. There are numerous apps and websites dedicated to supporting one another in the vegan community. If you're new to the vegan way of life, finding a support system to help with the transition is imperative.

Vegan restaurants and options available in traditional dining establishments are making it easier to dine with nonvegan friends and family. Eating a healthy vegan diet filled with nutritious foods still requires planning and some creativity. It will be difficult and expensive to adhere to this diet if you don't plan to cook and prepare most of your foods at home.

A plethora of vegan-friendly products have surfaced in the marketplace. Look at online recipe databases for new recipes, or reinvent your favorite dishes using new ingredients available on the market. Follow the same basic principles of meal planning by ensuring your plate contains proteins, whole grains, fruits, and vegetables. Use caution when balancing carbohydrates with protein and good sources of fat.

The Raw Food Diet

The belief that cooking foods destroys key nutrients is the theory behind raw food diets. Most individuals who follow a raw food diet are also vegan; however, some may choose to eat raw animal products like raw milk, cheese, sushi, and meat. Grains may also be consumed raw and the majority of calories will be from nuts, seeds, fruits, and vegetables.

Eating only raw foods is not a new way of life. The theory of eating only raw food dates back to the 1800s, yet there haven't been any scientifically reviewed studies supporting its claims. Foodborne illness is a serious concern when consuming raw milk and meat. In addition, following a highly restrictive diet can also have consequences to long-term health.

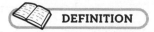 **DEFINITION**

Raw milk comes from cows, sheep, or goats, and has not undergone any of the conventional forms of pasteurization to kill potentially harmful bacteria. According to the U.S. Food and Drug Administration (FDA), pasteurization doesn't lower the milk's nutritional value and doesn't increase the potential for allergic reactions.

Adding the complexity of consuming only raw foods to an already challenging diet can be overwhelming for a beginner. This is a difficult and inconvenient diet for the average person. Foods need to be dehydrated, juiced, and blended to make food combinations.

The Juicing Diet

Many juicing diets are also considered "detox" diets. A juicing diet requires purchasing juice or using a machine to juice fruits and vegetables. Juice has generally the same vitamins, minerals, and phytonutrients as the raw fruits and vegetables. However, depending on the process used to obtain the juice, some of the nutrients may be reduced. Juice contains no fiber; it's removed in the processing of the fruits and vegetables.

There are various methods of following a juicing diet. Some people juice and drink one glass a day, or the juice is added to smoothies with Greek yogurt or peanut butter. The less restrictive forms are easier to follow for an extended length of time and won't leave you as nutritionally deficient. Following a restrictive juicing diet for an extended length of time will leave you deficient in protein, fiber, and fat.

Proponents tout the need to cleanse and detox your body by juicing. One of the primary jobs of the kidneys and liver is to filter out toxins. There's no scientific evidence to support claims that the juice diet's detoxing or cleansing contributes to good health.

Juicing can be healthy in small amounts. If you would rather drink your seven servings of vegetables than chew them, then by all means juice. However, remember you're missing out on all the fiber those fruits and vegetables would have provided. Eating whole vegetables and fruits will make you feel full. Not only will the fiber add bulk, but the process of chewing and swallowing also produces satiety.

Therapeutic Lifestyle Changes (TLC) Diet

Endorsed by the American Heart Association as a heart-healthy diet, the TLC diet was developed by the National Institutes of Health (NIH) to lower the risk of heart disease and cholesterol.

Giving up high-fat foods to keep your total fat intake between 25 and 35 percent of your daily calories is an important factor in the TLC diet. Trans fat should be eliminated and saturated fat should be kept to less than 7 percent of your daily calories (for a 2,000-calorie diet this equates to less than 13g per day). To help with the modifications, the TLC diet suggests including whole nuts instead of nut butter, swapping out butter for heart-healthy oils, and eliminating fried foods. Reducing dietary cholesterol to less than 200mg per day is also advised.

Calorie targets are based on your personal goals, such as lowering your low-density lipoprotein (LDL), the bad cholesterol, or losing weight. Increasing fiber-rich foods to help bind cholesterol in the blood is key.

Items to focus on:

- 3-5 servings of vegetables and beans

- 2-4 servings of fruits

- 6+ servings of whole grains

- 2-3 servings of low-fat and nonfat dairy

- 5 oz. of lean protein (skinless chicken breast or turkey)

- 2 meals per week of high omega-3 fish

- 30 minutes a day of physical activity

- Supplementing with a daily multivitamin

For those who don't see a reduction in their cholesterol or their level is still higher than acceptable, they should add:

- 5-10g of soluble fiber (oats, whole fruits, or beans)

- 2-3g of plant sterols/stanols

You should also reduce or eliminate:

- Red meat (high saturated fat content)

- Alcohol

- Simple sugar

- Sodium intake to less than 2,300mg per day

To learn to be successful on the TLC diet, you'll need to master reading food labels, which include a lot of key information for the TLC dieter. By reading the labels, you can determine the total amounts of saturated and trans fats. Cholesterol and fiber amounts are also included on the labels. By continuously reading labels, you'll become proficient in determining if a food has added sugar or if the sodium content is in line with your intake.

FOODIE FACTOID

Sterols and stanols are found naturally in some plants. Eating them has been shown to help lower cholesterol in your bloodstream by blocking the absorption of LDL in your small intestine and preventing the cholesterol from blocking your arteries. While they do occur naturally in small amounts, they're also being added to foods. Getting plant sterols/stanols from whole foods is the best approach. However, if you have high cholesterol or have had a heart attack, eating 2 to 3g per day from whole and fortified foods has been shown to lower your LDL by 6 to 15 percent.

If you dine out, you'll also need to become proficient at navigating nutritional information provided by restaurants. Cooking at home also will be essential to being successful on the TLC diet. Even though the diet may increase your intake of fruits and vegetables, a reduction in meat and eliminating processed foods will offset the cost at the grocery store and may even save you money.

Dietary Approaches to Stop Hypertension (DASH) Diet

Designed to lower blood pressure, the DASH diet is based in science. It's a commonsense approach to changing the way you eat. You don't need to have hypertension (high blood pressure) to follow this diet. It has many health benefits and touts weight loss as a possible side effect. The DASH diet helps with weight loss mainly because you're giving up daily splurges of high-calorie, fat-filled processed foods. The DASH diet helps you determine the number of calories you need based on your height, weight, and activity levels. The basic premise is a reduction in saturated and trans fat, cholesterol, sodium, and refined sugar. It increases your intake of foods high in potassium, calcium, magnesium, protein, and fiber.

Daily and weekly goals for a 2,000-calorie diet are:

- 4-5 servings of fruit (per day)

- 4-5 servings of vegetables (per day)

- 6-8 servings of whole grains (per day)

- 2-3 servings of fat-free or low-fat dairy (per day)

- 2-3 servings of heart-healthy oils (per day)

- 6 oz. of lean protein (no more than 4 egg yolks per week)

- 4-5 servings of nuts and seeds per week

- Less than 5 servings of sweets per week

- Two meatless meals per week

- Reduce sodium to 2,300mg with a goal of under 1,500mg (per day)

- 30 minutes of physical activity each day

- Replace salt with herbs, spices, salt-free blends, lemon juice, and vinegars (per day)

This diet has been proven to lower LDL and triglycerides and increase HDL. The DASH diet is similar to the Mediterranean diet (but without the red wine and additional servings of heart-healthy fats). There's a vegetarian version of the diet for those who choose not to eat meat. Alcohol also is limited.

The DASH diet is designed as a long-term lifestyle change, making it very easy to stay on for quite some time. There are no special foods to buy and once you get accustomed to the recommended components, it will be easier to eat out. You'll likely need to ask for substitutions at restaurants, such as no sauce on the chicken and fresh fruit instead of fries.

NOTABLE INSIGHT

Reducing your sodium intake can be a real challenge. The average American consumes 4,000 to 5,000 milligrams per day, with recommendations of only 1,500 to 2,300 milligrams per day depending on your health needs. Fresh vegetables are a smart choice, but frozen and canned can be good options, too. Just be sure to read the labels and if you purchase canned, look for those with no added salt or reduced sodium. Rinsing your canned veggies will also lower the sodium levels. Use salt-free spice blends or make your own. Flavored sauces, rice, canned soups, deli meats, and processed foods are particularly high in salt. Look for items with less than 450mg per serving.

The Paleo Diet

Our ancestors were hunters and gatherers 100,000 years ago. It was a preagricultural era, which means they didn't have cultivated crops or farmed animals—no dairy, wheat, oats, or legumes. Everything consumed was gathered from the land or hunted.

Incorporating the hunter-gatherer philosophy into our modern-day diet eliminates all processed foods, salt, refined sugars, alcohol, grains (wheat, oats, and quinoa), starchy vegetable (potatoes, sweet potatoes, and squash), legumes, dairy, and animals raised on grain. While many Paleo dieters tout it as a high-protein diet, its guidelines for protein, carbohydrate, and fats are close to the acceptable macronutrient distribution range (AMDR).

Individuals who follow the Paleolithic diet eat meat (grass-fed only), fish, chicken, eggs, nuts, and seeds, along with high amounts of nonstarchy fruits and vegetables. The glycemic index is also taken into consideration when choosing foods. Fruits and vegetables with high sugar contents (grapes, bananas, and watermelon) are eaten infrequently. The acid-base balance is a component of the Paleo diet. Dieters believe balancing foods that raise (meats) or lower (fruits and vegetables) the pH of your blood will lead to better health.

Following the Paleo diet long-term may be tricky and expensive. The cost of eating large amounts of grass-fed meats (beef, wild boar, bison, and wild game) with fresh fruits and vegetables can add up quickly. Eating out can be difficult unless you frequent higher-end establishments that offer grass-fed meats.

 FOODIE FACTOID

According to researchers at Texas A&M, the fatty acid profile of grass-fed beef and grain-finished beef are mostly monounsaturated and saturated fats. Beef from cows fed longer on grain may have more monounsaturated fat, which may lower cholesterol. Grass-fed beef may have a slightly higher (.02 grams versus .055 grams) omega-3 fatty acid level. Daily requirements for women are 1.1g and for men 1.6g.

This diet has healthy components, such as reduced salt intake and elimination of refined sugars, soda, and sports drinks. The elimination of grains and dairy, however, could lead to deficiencies in many B vitamins and calcium. Ensure plenty of calcium rich vegetables are in your diet and consider supplementing with B vitamins. Also, be aware that coffee is *not* on the Paleo diet!

Commercial Diet Plans

In 2014, weight-loss companies brought in over $2.5 billion. With that kind of revenue generated, you should expect big results. Studies show some of the top companies do succeed in assisting clients with weight loss, but the success generally is short term.

The plans that focus on portion control tend to have the best results. Costs of the plans range from $40 to over $700 a month, depending on the level of support, participation, and amount of food purchased. Commercial diet plans aren't for everyone. But for someone who needs or wants continued support, they're a viable option.

Weight Watchers

The Weight Watchers approach to weight loss is commercially endorsed by highly paid starlets featuring striking differences between their before and after photos. This program is based on the principle that no two calories are created equal.

The program assigns points to foods based on how long they'll fill you up. Lower-point foods will make you feel fuller longer. Higher-point foods are quick used. The key is sticking to your points and learning how to choose foods, which will help keep the weight off. No foods are off limits, just higher in points. Fresh fruits and vegetables are free, so eat away. Weight Watchers claims eating out is easy with a few simple points, and some restaurants even have Weight Watcher points printed on their menus. Points are sufficient to allow for three meals and two snacks daily.

Research shows programs offering emotional support and group sessions lead to better compliance. This philosophy is taken to heart at Weight Watchers. A smartphone app is available to help you count points as you go; it includes activity tracking, recipes, customized meals, videos, a support community, and a 24/7 help line for continuous support.

Personal coaches are also available to connect one-on-one via phone or email as often as you want. You also can sign up to receive text reminders and motivation from your coach. There are a variety of fees associated with belonging to Weight Watchers and for additional benefits, such as unlimited group sessions and personal coaching.

The Weight Watcher's plan was originally designed for people to prepare their own fresh foods at home. However, Weight Watchers now has an entire line of prepackaged and pre-portioned meals available to choose from in your local grocery store.

Due to calorie restriction, Weight Watchers recommends taking a daily multivitamin to ensure an adequate intake of calcium, zinc, magnesium, iron, and B_{12}.

Jenny Craig

Another weight loss company using high profile, well-paid actors, Jenny Craig prides itself on personalizing a diet plan for you. It provides all the foods you need for your meals, simplifying the process of meal preparation.

The program follows guidelines set out as a plan for you using your weight loss goals, fitness habits, motivation level, and current weight. Jenny Craig emphasizes an active lifestyle along with behavior modification and calorie reduction.

On Jenny Craig you'll eat three meals, two snacks, and one dessert daily. The pre-portioned meals are small but nutritionally balanced. The types of foods provided are designed to help you feel full as long as possible. Fresh fruit and low-fat dairy are also included. Gluten-free meals are also offered.

Financially, you'll have to purchase all the premade meals and snacks until you're halfway to your weight loss goal. If you have a family, you'll still have to cook regular meals for them, as the foods provided only feed one. In the beginning, there's limited flexibility for dining out or eating at a friend's house. An event such as a party or outing where food is central becomes difficult. These factors may affect your ability to stay on the diet long term.

A monthly fee is associated with the program and builds in a weekly consultation to discuss your progress. The consultant will offer advice to you on the phone or in person.

The program has no ending point, and some stay on it for years while slowly incorporating their own home-cooked meals. Jenny Craig admits it's challenging to get enough of all nutrients on a low-calorie program and recommends taking a multivitamin.

Atkins

Well known for the high-protein, low-carb diet, Atkins was developed by a cardiologist. This diet incorporates four levels of carbohydrate intake with the goal of putting your body into ketosis (a state in which your body no longer has glycogen to use as fuel for the brain and has to convert fat into fuel, creating ketones as a byproduct). The problem with ketosis is your brain is not happy; it prefers glycogen as its source of fuel. You may experience weakness, nausea, bad breath, constipation (there's very little fiber in the diet), and being downright cranky. The ketones in the blood also cause inflammation.

Some studies have shown weight loss and improved waist circumference. However, it's possible the weight loss comes from reducing calories rather than the actual types of foods you eat. One study did report weight loss of approximately 10 pounds in 1 year of Atkins participants. But it also reported the participants ate higher levels of carbohydrates than were outlined by the diet.

As for the nutritional side effects of the diet, sodium exceeds the recommended amount, and it will be difficult to get nutrients readily available in grains, such as fiber and B vitamins. With limited dairy in the first phases, it's a good idea to supplement with calcium. The diet is extremely high in fat, with the intake well over the AMDR and carbohydrate intake far under. It's safe to say the Atkins plan does not provide a well-balanced diet.

It can be an expensive diet to follow due to the amount of meat required, and especially if you purchase the Atkins food products. Frozen meals are available in select stores, and protein bars, shakes, and treats can be purchased in stores or online. The Atkins website offers free online weight loss tools, such as a carb tracker, recipes, meal plans, shopping lists, forums, and chat groups. There's also a smartphone app available. The diet is difficult to stick to long term with its rigorous restrictions on carbohydrates. Eating bacon may sound like fun for a while, but it can get old quickly. Imagine no baked potatoes, breadless sandwiches, and meatballs without pasta.

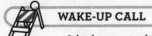

WAKE-UP CALL

A high-protein diet should never be followed if you have kidney disease or renal insufficiency. The American Diabetes Association (ADA) doesn't recommend a high-protein diet to aid in weight loss.

South Beach

The premise of this diet is lower carbs, higher protein, and more healthy fat than the typical American diet. You toss out the unrefined carbs and bad fats, and replace them with whole grain carbs and healthy fats. That sounds pretty reasonable, right?

Be cautioned, the diet can be pretty restrictive in the early phases, but it does allow for three meals, two snacks, and a dessert each day. Phase one starts out highly restrictive but eases up as you progress. Vegetables, lean protein (chicken, fish, and turkey), nuts, and eggs are the mainstays of the diet. Whole grains, fruits, and additional vegetables are added in the second phase. The final phase is where you maintain your weight and theoretically stay there for the rest of your life. This stage has no "off-limits" foods, but has limits on certain items such as "good fats." Once you get to the maintenance phase, the diet is a fairly well-rounded, healthy meal plan. Add some extra nutrients by incorporating fruits and vegetables high in antioxidants and vitamins and minerals.

The prescribed menus can be expensive, but tweaking the meals to stay within the confines of the diet will help save some money at the grocery store. There are specific South Beach products you can purchase in select stores or have delivered to your home. Offerings include meals and a wide variety of bars (including gluten-free).

South Beach offers a mobile app as well as online interactive tools, recipes, meal plans, coaching, and a support community.

The Least You Need to Know

- You can lose weight on any diet. It's the long-term changes in your eating habits and lifestyle that keep the weight off.
- Diets that focus on eating whole foods will provide you with the best variety of nutrients.
- Going vegetarian requires thoughtfully planned meals to make certain your body doesn't miss out on important nutrients like vitamin B12, vitamin D, and calcium.
- Successful dieters are actively involved in their food choices and leave no meals to chance.

Superfoods: Are They Real or Just Good Marketing Tactics?

Have you ever wondered if foods really have superpowers? Well, there are many nutrient-packed foods that just might. Their value comes not from anything added to them but from just what Mother Nature provides.

In this chapter, we'll find out exactly what the term "super-foods" means and discover the many benefits these powerful foods provide for our physical and mental health. Many of the foods we'll discuss are known to boost strength and energy, help prevent disease, and keep us living healthier and longer.

In This Chapter

- What exactly constitutes a "superfood?"
- What superfoods can do for you
- What foods are considered superfoods and why
- How to incorporate superfoods into your daily diet

What Makes a Food Super?

Most of the time the term "superfood" is more of a marketing term than a true label claim. However, this term does still carry some merit. The problem is that it's not a technical definition, so companies are at liberty to label nearly anything a superfood. So it's buyer beware when you purchase a packaged food product or supplement that is labeled a superfood!

The foods we'll discuss are not packaged as superfoods, but are considered super due to the wide array of nutrients they naturally contain. There's no one single food that contains all the phyto-nutrients, antioxidants, vitamins, minerals, fiber, and so on your body requires on a daily basis for good health and to fight disease. Almost every food in the produce section is a superfood in some way, whether it's categorized that way or not. Your best bet is to eat a variety of fresh and wholesome foods daily to get the nutrients you need to stay healthy and feel your best.

Superfoods and Their Benefits

There are many healthy foods that have never been called "super." However, certain foods are deemed superfoods because they're nutrient powerhouses that pack large doses of antioxidants, *polyphenols,* phytonutrients, vitamins, minerals, and more in a fairly small serving. Including them daily in a healthy and well-balanced diet may help to reduce your risk for chronic disease, prolong your life, and support better overall health.

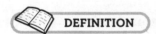 **DEFINITION**

> **Polyphenols** are micronutrients found in certain foods that act as powerful antioxidants. Studies have proven that polyphenols can help to prevent degenerative diseases, such as cancer and heart disease, as well as reduce the effects of aging.

Longevity

One of the benefits to consuming superfoods, and healthier foods in general, is that they lower the risk for both chronic disease and age-related diseases. Research has found groups of people around the world who live longer and enjoy healthier lives due to the foods they regularly include in their diets.

Mental Health

When we discuss mental health, we're talking about a whole host of issues ranging from depression and anxiety to dementia and Alzheimer's disease. Food matters when it comes to your brain power and mental health. Although some mental health issues can be genetic, your overall lifestyle can still help lower your risk for these mental disorders and sometimes help manage them once you have them. Not only can true mental disorders be affected by nutrition, but your everyday mood can also be affected by the foods you eat, and vice versa. In fact, a diet high in sugar and processed foods has been linked to depression. For or many people, when they get depressed or stressed they turn to emotional eating and consume more processed foods that are high in sugar. It becomes a vicious cycle that needs to be broken.

Dementia and Alzheimer's disease are not a natural part of aging. For many of these debilitating and deadly mental sufferers, the major factors were lifestyle and the foods they generally ate during their lifetime. Of course, genetics and medical history also play a part, but lifestyle and diet are also a large piece of the picture. There's no one superfood or even a handful of superfoods that can guarantee good mental health, but generally eating a healthier diet and exercising on a regular basis will go a long way toward lowering your risk.

Energy

Food is our number one source of energy. However, you must consume the right foods to attain the energy your body truly needs. Much of society is accustomed to consuming unhealthy diets, which provide minimal energy levels. Many people don't even realize how much better they could feel and how much more energy they could have by simply eating a healthier diet. Lower energy levels can greatly affect everyday life, including the motivation to exercise and stay active, which in turn can affect health and mood.

When people consume unhealthy diets and feel exhausted, they turn to more unhealthy foods and beverages containing sugar and caffeine to give them the boost they need for their energy reserves. Again, it becomes a vicious cycle that needs to be broken. Not only does their low energy affect the way they feel both physically and mentally, but it wreaks havoc on their immune system as well, leaving them more susceptible to illness, depression, and even chronic conditions such as heart disease.

 NOTABLE INSIGHT

Proper nutrition and the timing of what you eat can make all the difference, making you feel alert and powerful. It provides you with the energy you need to be physically active, think clearly, and feel positive. Shoot for eating three healthy meals a day with portion-controlled healthy snacks in between for all-day energy.

A Healthy Sex Drive

Nutritional deficiencies from not eating properly can also have an impact on your libido. Essentially, what's good for your heart is also good for your sex drive. A low sex drive doesn't have to be a part of normal aging. With proper nutrition and a healthier lifestyle, you can achieve a normal libido at any age. Without you even realizing it, the unhealthy foods you're eating may be contributing to a low sex drive. You might feel it's simply part of the aging process, but it's simply not. Proper nutrition, including superfoods, and a healthy lifestyle can make an immense difference in your sex drive.

Examples of Superfoods

You should be sure to make the following superfoods a regular part of your healthy diet. While this section doesn't discuss all the superfoods that exist, it will give you a good place to start. The key is to eat a variety of healthy foods so you receive a wide variety of nutrients.

Dark Chocolate

Lucky for us that dark chocolate is considered a superfood! Yum! But there is more to dark chocolate than just its creamy, melt-in-your-mouth goodness. Dark chocolate is made from cocoa beans that are chockfull of polyphenols and antioxidants and rich in flavonoids. Flavonoids help protect plants from environmental toxins and help repair cell damage. The great news is that it appears we, too, get these same benefits when we eat flavonoid-containing foods such as dark chocolate, fruits, and vegetables.

Flavanols are the main type of flavonoid found in cocoa and dark chocolate. In addition to their powerful antioxidant properties, flavanols may benefit vascular health by lowering blood pressure and improving blood flow to the brain and the heart, thus reducing the risk for heart attack and stroke. Other benefits of flavanols include acting as an anti-inflammatory and lowering the risk for cognitive impairment and certain cancers.

Other foods rich in flavanols include cranberries and other specific berries, apples, pomegranates, peanuts, onions, tea, and red wine. Keep in mind that even though dark chocolate may have some amazing health benefits, you should eat it in moderation and look for 70 percent cacao in the chocolate. Most commercial chocolate has not only raw cocoa but added fat, sugar, and calories.

Here are some ways to enjoy dark chocolate:

- Add plain cocoa powder to low-fat or fat-free milk.
- Grate dark chocolate over fresh fruit or smoothies.
- Add grated dark chocolate to savory sauces.

- Add dark chocolate chips to oatmeal.
- Mix chocolate into low-fat Greek yogurt.

 FOODIE FACTOID

If you want to add all of the amazing health benefits of dark chocolate without the added fats and sugar, you need to select a product containing least 70 percent cacao. The darker the chocolate, the less sugar it will contain.

Berries

Berries are at the top of the list as far as superfoods go. There's a vast variety to choose from, including blueberries, blackberries, cranberries, strawberries, and raspberries, just to name just a few. If you want to get a little more exotic, there are açai berries and goji berries.

Berries are packed with disease-fighting phytochemicals, including anthocyanins, another part of the flavonoid family of polyphenols. These powerful compounds have antioxidant properties that studies suggest help to reduce the risk of cardiovascular disease (CVD), cognitive decline, and cancer. These red and blue fruits can also help boost your immunity and are anti-inflammatory.

When choosing berries, the darker they are, the more disease-fighting antioxidants they contain. Shoot for a serving of some variety of berries daily. Fresh is great, but frozen are just as good if they're out of season.

Here are some ways to enjoy berries:

- Put berries on your morning cereal (cold or hot).
- Add them to low-fat yogurt—layer them with yogurt to create a parfait for a yummy and snappy-looking dessert.
- Add them to smoothies. (Using frozen berries gives your smoothie a thicker consistency.)
- Enjoy them plain or mixed with other fruits in a fruit salad.
- Sprinkle them over your favorite salad.

Kale

Kale is a super-healthy green, actually a member of the cabbage family, and falls under the heading of cruciferous vegetables. Kale isn't the only cruciferous vegetable that's super-healthy. Others include cabbage, broccoli, cauliflower, collard greens, and brussels sprouts.

Kale is very nutrient-dense and loaded with a wide array of nutrients, including vitamins A, K, C, and B6, manganese, calcium, copper, potassium, and magnesium. Kale also contains fiber and very little fat, but the fat it does have is an omega-3 fatty acid.

Kale is loaded with all types of beneficial compounds that have tremendous health benefits. Two of these include quercetin and kaempferol, both of which provide heart protection and lower blood pressure, and have anti-inflammatory, antiviral, antidepressant, and anticancer effects. In addition, kale is high in lutein and zeaxanthin, antioxidants that are linked to good eye health.

Here are some ways to enjoy kale:

- Steam kale plain as a side dish.

- Use thinly sliced raw kale in salads.

- Make kale chips by brushing with extra virgin olive oil, sprinkling on a little salt, and baking until crisp.

- Mix kale with brown rice or whole-grain pasta.

 FOODIE FACTOID

Kale is not really high in vitamin A itself, but it's an excellent source of beta-carotene, an antioxidant that turns into vitamin A in the body.

Chia Seeds

Chia seeds are tiny black seeds that come from the chia plant, which is native to Mexico and Guatemala. These seeds are rich sources of insoluble fiber and omega-3 fatty acids in the form of alpha-linolenic acid (ALA). Chia seeds are one of the best-known plant sources of omega-3 fatty acids, even higher in these healthy fats than flaxseeds. In addition, they provide high-quality protein (meaning they contain all of the essential amino acids) and loads of essential minerals and antioxidants such as manganese, phosphorus, copper, selenium, copper, magnesium, and calcium.

Chia seeds may improve risk factors for both heart disease and diabetes and improve digestive health.

Here are some ways to enjoy chia seeds:

- Add chia seeds to baked goods.

- Sprinkle chia seeds on cold or hot cereal.

- Mix chia seeds in your oatmeal.

- Top your low-fat yogurt with chia seeds.

- Mix chia seeds in your vegetable or rice dishes.

 WAKE-UP CALL

In large doses, chia seeds can have blood-thinning effects. If you're taking blood-thinning medications, consult with your doctor before incorporating these seeds into your diet. Chia seeds also contain a plant compound called phytic acid, which can combine with minerals such as iron and zinc and inhibit their absorption.

Pomegranates

Pomegranates are one healthy fruit. They're classified as part of the berry family, but look more like a red apple with a funny stem. Their skin is very thick and inedible, but inside are hundreds of sweet edible seeds called arils. These arils are the part of the fruit people eat, either raw or processed into juice.

Pomegranates sport an impressive nutritional profile starting with 7 grams of fiber per 1 cup of arils. They also contain protein, vitamin C, vitamin K, folate, and potassium. There are two plant compounds in pomegranates that are responsible for most of their amazing health benefits: punicalagins and punicic acid. Punicalagins are very powerful antioxidants found mainly in the juice and peel of the fruit. Punicic acid, sometimes called pomegranate seed oil, is the main fatty acid found in the arils.

Pomegranates have anti-inflammatory effects, help fight against prostate and breast cancer, may lower blood pressure, help alleviate arthritis and joint pain, lower your risk of heart disease, help improve memory, and improve exercise performance. And if that isn't enough, pomegranates also have antibacterial and antiviral properties, which may help against common gum diseases.

Here are some ways to enjoy pomegranates:

- Add pomegranate seeds to low-fat vanilla yogurt.

- Try pomegranate juice as an alternative beverage.

- Juice the seeds and use them as a marinade on chicken, fish, shrimp, or pork.

- Toss pomegranate seeds on salads.

- Eat them as a snack.

Black Beans

Beans are one of the key food groups for preventing disease and optimizing health. The Dietary Guidelines for Americans recommends consuming at least 3 cups of *legumes* or beans weekly. When it comes to beans, black beans top the list and provide a good source of molybdenum, folate, fiber, copper, and magnesium.

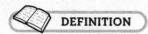 **DEFINITION**

> **Legumes** are a class of vegetable and include not only beans but peas and lentils as well.

All beans in general are a winning combination of high-quality carbs, lean protein, and soluble fiber, which helps to stabilize blood sugar levels and keep hunger in check. In addition, they aid your digestive tract and provide cardiovascular benefits. Black beans are chockfull of an impressive array of antioxidant and anti-inflammatory phytonutrients.

Beans are very inexpensive, versatile, and even fat-free. You can buy them dried or canned. When using canned beans, rinse them thoroughly to lower the sodium content. Besides black beans, other great varieties of legumes that provide as many health benefits include chickpeas, lentils, kidney beans, soybeans, navy beans, and pinto beans.

Here are some ways to enjoy black beans:

- Add the beans to chili, casseroles, and soups.

- Toss beans in your salad.

- Use them to make a hummus-style dip.

- Use them as a stuffing for tacos and/or burritos.

- Toss beans with brown rice and salsa for a quick, nutritious side dish.

- Use them with guacamole as a layered dip for veggies.

Salmon

Salmon and other fatty fish (such as lake trout, sardines, herring, albacore tuna, and mackerel) are a great source of lean high-quality protein, contain no saturated fat, and are an excellent concentrated source of omega-3 fatty acids. Salmon provides omega-3 fatty acids in the form of eicosapentaenoic acid (EPA) and docosahexaenoic acid (DHA). Salmon is also an excellent source of vitamin B_{12}, vitamin D, selenium, niacin, and phosphorus.

EPA and DHA omega-3 fatty acids are known to reduce the risk for diabetes; increase the effectiveness of insulin; support joint cartilage; support eye health; be anti-inflammatory; and decrease the risk for heart disease, some types of cancer, Alzheimer's disease, and other cognitive issues.

The goal should be to include at least 7 ounces of fatty fish, such as salmon, in your diet each week.

Here are some ways to enjoy salmon:

- Grill it.

- Use cold salmon in a salad.

- Make "salmon burgers."

- Use salmon to make fish tacos.

- Add it to a chowder-based soup.

Turmeric

Turmeric is an Indian spice that comes from the root of the *curcuma longa* plant, which is a relative to ginger root. Best known as a main ingredient in curry, tumeric's deep yellow-orange color is also what gives mustard its bright yellow color.

The pigment that gives turmeric its yellow-orange color is called *curcumin*, which is believed to be the primary component that contributes to its amazing health benefits as well as its powerful antioxidant properties. Curcumin has been found to provide anti-inflammatory effects, be an effective treatment for inflammatory bowel disease (IBD), provide relieve for arthritis sufferers, improve liver function, offer protection from cardiovascular disease, lower cholesterol, lower the risk of Alzheimer's disease, and help prevent some types of cancer.

You can enjoy turmeric by using it in your daily meal plan. Turmeric is also available in powdered capsule form. The general recommendation is 400 to 600mg three times per day of a standardized powder (curcumin). Be patient, as it may take up to a few months before full benefits take place. You shouldn't use turmeric supplements if you have gallstones or bile duct dysfunction. Speak with your doctor before using a turmeric supplement if you have diabetes, are pregnant, on a blood-thinning medication, and/or on medication to reduce stomach acid.

Here are some ways to enjoy turmeric in your daily diet:

- Mix it with brown rice for a side dish.

- Add it to egg salad or deviled eggs.

- Add it to salad dressings.

- Use turmeric as a spice to flavor lentils and beans.

- Add it to spice up and add color to white cauliflower.

Walnuts

Who doesn't like a handful of walnuts, pistachios, cashews, pecans, or macadamia nuts? All of these are part of the tree nut family. It only takes a very small amount daily, 1 ounce in fact, to provide significant health benefits. In the case of walnuts, that equals about seven whole shelled nuts.

Besides tasting yummy, walnuts are a rich source of heart-healthy monounsaturated fats as well as omega-3 fatty acids in the form of alpha-linolenic (ALA). Walnuts are best consumed in their whole form, including the skin. Researchers are convinced the skin contains the vast majority of the polyphenols, which are micronutrients that act as powerful antioxidants. Walnuts offer cardiovascular benefits, reduce issues in metabolic syndrome, provide significant benefits for those with type 2 diabetes, and can help lower the risk for certain cancers. But keep in mind that as healthy as they are, nuts are also considered a fat—though a healthy fat—and a little bit packs in lots of calories, so be mindful of your portion size.

Here are some ways to enjoy walnuts:

- Sprinkle them on salads.

- Eat them as a snack.

- Use them to make a pesto.

- Sprinkle them on top of oatmeal or yogurt.

- Mix walnuts in with chicken, tuna, or curried turkey salads.

Avocados

Did you know that avocados are part of the fruit family? They're a nutritional gem rich in heart-healthy monounsaturated fats—one of the healthiest fats around. They're also a good source of fiber; potassium; vitamins C and K, folate, and B6, just to name just a few.

In addition, avocados help reduce excess cholesterol, triglyceride levels, and inflammation; benefit heart health; combat cancer cells, and help to protect the liver. The fat in avocados also helps to increase absorption of antioxidants from other foods you eat. In addition, they contain two antioxidants, lutein and zeaxanthin, both of which are incredibly essential for good eye health.

Here are some ways to enjoy avocados:

- Add sliced avocado to sandwiches, chicken, or burgers.

- Use them to make guacamole dip.

- Dice them up and mix with chopped tomatoes and onions along with a pinch of salt and pepper and use as a side dish.

- Toss cubed avocado into a salad or pasta salad.

 NOTABLE INSIGHT

Avocados are high in potassium, which is an important mineral that is lacking in the diets of the majority of Americans.

Sample Superfoods Recipe

Wilted Kale Salad

Yield:	Prep Time:	Cook Time:	
4 servings	15 minutes	1 minute	
Nutrition Facts for one serving:			
440 calories	28g total fat	4.5g saturated fat	50mg cholesterol
250mg sodium	30g carbohydrates	5g fiber	21g protein

Dressing:

3 TB. extra virgin olive oil

1 TB. balsamic vinegar

1 TB. agave nectar

$^1/_8$ tsp. salt

Ingredients:

1 TB. olive oil

1 bunch lacinato kale

$^1/_8$ tsp. kosher salt

8 oz. salmon, grilled and chilled

1 pear, diced

$^3/_4$ cup pomegranate seeds

$^1/_4$ cup feta cheese

$^1/_4$ cup walnuts, chopped and toasted

1. Make the dressing by whisking the olive oil, vinegar, agave, and salt in a small mixing bowl. Set aside.

2. Stack the kale leaves into manageable stacks and slice into $1/4$-inch strips. Discard the stems or save for another use.

3. Heat oil in a large skillet over medium heat. Add kale and cook for 1 minute. Immediately remove from heat and transfer to a mixing bowl.

4. Combine salad dressing, kosher salt with kale. Mix well.

5. Plate each salad individually. Begin with a layer of wilted kale, 2 ounces salmon, 2 tablespoons pear, 1 tablespoon pomegranate seeds, 1 tablespoon feta cheese, and 1 tablespoon walnuts.

Cook's note: Substitute other nuts such as pine nuts, pecans, cashews, or sliced almonds to change up your meal.

The Least You Need to Know

- Recognizing superfoods will help aid you in eating a nutrition-packed diet.
- Superfoods come from every food group.
- Superfoods have numerous health benefits, including aiding your sex drive as you age.
- If there's a healthy superfood you haven't tried, do it now. Don't be afraid to explore and try something new. You may even find you have a new favorite food that also benefits your health.

CHAPTER

22

Controversial Foods

When it comes to controversial foods, what makes the headlines and travels the media circuit is king. Unfortunately, the original story may get exaggerated or be taken out of context, often leaving the consumer bewildered as to what to believe. Some foods are considered to be controversial because they're not grown sustainably, and others are controversial due to the handling and treatment of animals as well as their impact on the environment.

In this chapter, we'll explore the facts surrounding controversial foods and beverages such as coffee and wine, and whether or not they should be included in your diet.

Why Certain Foods Are Considered Controversial

Oftentimes there is some grain of truth behind food controversies. Different sources pick up one side of a story and expand upon it without looking into the full background and illuminating the truth. However, by then it's too late and the food controversy is blown completely out of proportion. It's best you do your own research about these controversial foods and make your own decisions about the foods to include in your diet.

Eggs

Purchasing eggs at your local market can be overwhelming. Key words such as *cage-free*, *free-range*, *all-natural*, and *hormone-free* are labeled on the cartons, but what do they really mean and how do you make the right choice?

Eggs are big business. According to the U.S. Department of Agriculture (USDA), approximately 8 billion eggs a month produced by over 360 million laying hens in the United States. Consumer concerns have surfaced regarding the hens' living conditions and how humanely they're treated. Many people envision hens packed into tight, filthy cages that breed disease. Consumers also believe it's common practice to use high amounts of antibiotics to keep production levels high.

According to the USDA, federal law prohibits the use of all hormones when raising any kind of poultry. Antibiotics are used only when hens are ill. There are also specific guidelines for antibiotic withdrawal. During that period, the layers' eggs are not allowed to enter the market.

> **WAKE-UP CALL**
>
> The Cleveland Clinic reports only about 20 percent of the cholesterol in your blood comes from foods in your diet. The Harvard School of Public Health states the biggest factor in your diet is the combination and types of carbohydrates and fats consumed. Eliminating trans fats and reducing foods high in saturated fat along with increasing high-fiber grains will have a bigger impact on your blood cholesterol levels than the cholesterol content in your food.

From a nutrition standpoint, eggs have been given a bad rap over the years due to their levels of dietary cholesterol. Eggs also have the potential to carry the bacteria salmonella, which is the most common cause of food poisoning in the United States. This bacterium resides inside the egg, typically in the yolk, although it can be present anywhere. According to the Centers for Disease Control and Prevention (CDC), only 1 in 10,000 eggs contains salmonella. This is why every restaurant that serves eggs puts a warning on the menu regarding consumption of undercooked eggs. Cooking the egg to an internal temperature of 160°F where the yolk and white are firm reduces the risk by killing any bacteria present. Most health experts agree that certain people shouldn't consume undercooked eggs, such as the very young or old and those with a compromised immune system.

The Hen House

How do you know if the eggs you're purchasing come from a source that provides a healthy, humane, safe living environment for the chickens? Understanding the industry lingo can help guide you to the right place to spend your dollars. According to the American Egg Board, there are no regulations in the egg industry defining cage-free or free roaming. Generally, these terms mean the animals are not held in cages; instead they roam freely in a barn or indoor sheltered area. While some may have access to the outdoors, there are no standards stating how much, if any, access should be provided. Layers have free access to food and water and are provided perches, nests, and floor space to allow them to engage in some natural behaviors. However, there is no third-party audit to ensure any of these procedures are followed.

Free-range or pasture-fed eggs come from hens with outdoor access determined by weather conditions, environmental concerns, and state laws. Often the layers forage for some of their food and eat a diet consisting of grains. Indoor perches and nesting areas are provided. Similar to cage-free, certified humane eggs come from hens housed in large barns or other types of indoor facility with no required outdoor access. These hens are allowed more natural behavior; however, *induced molting* is permitted as long as the elimination of food is not practiced. Antibiotics may not be used and the stocking density, or amount of hens per square foot, is specified. Third-party audits are performed to ensure the farms are following the correct procedures and policies.

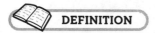 **DEFINITION**

> According to the American Egg board, **induced molting** is a commonly used practice in the egg industry. Hens are fed lower qualities of feed to induce a period when eggs will not be laid. At the end of this period, the hen's reproductive quality is revitalized, which enables the hens to produce a greater number of eggs. Organic farming practices prohibit the use of induced molting.

The molting process occurs naturally in hens once a year. Induced by the shortened days of autumn, hens will stop laying for a short period. However, with low stress, controlled temperatures, and artificially lit barns, hens can go a whole year without molting, which results in a decline in production and egg quality.

Utilizing an Enriched Colony System produces American Humane Certified eggs. This system allows for hens to have space for natural behavior, although their confinement space may be small. Eggs from the Enriched Colony System may come from layers caged or with free access. There's no way to know which housing method is used.

Family farms may specify their eggs are Animal Welfare approved. These layers have ongoing access to the outdoors, open pasture, and shelter. No antibiotics are allowed and their feed is vegetarian. Family farms do adhere to certain regulated standards. Many other labeled practices are not standardized or audited. Eggs labeled that the hens had vegetarian diets are not regulated. The term "natural eggs" also has no defined meaning. Eggs cannot be labeled antibiotic-free unless they're certified organic, and they have no regulation associated with them.

Certified organic eggs come from hens enclosed inside large barns. These hens are required to have access to the outdoors. However, there are no standards as to what "outdoor access" entails. Induced molting of all varieties is permitted, including complete food deprivation. Feed is 100 percent vegetarian and pesticide-free, and layers are not allowed to receive antibiotics.

Chicken feed is scientifically balanced to provide optimal health for the layer and to produce the best quality eggs. Hens have continuous access to water, and feed is dispensed at timed intervals. All feed additives have been proven to be safe for hens and consumers. Additives may consist of antioxidants, omega-3s, and mold inhibitors to maintain feed quality.

Cholesterol and Fat

"The Incredible Edible Egg," a tagline used by the American Egg Board, sums up the nutritional makeup of the egg. High in biologically available protein, the egg is relativity inexpensive compared to other protein foods ounce per ounce. An egg is comprised of two main edible parts: the white and the yolk.

The white consists of approximately two thirds of the volume of the egg with 17 calories and just over half the egg's total protein. It also contains no fat and the majority of the egg's niacin, riboflavin, magnesium, potassium, and sodium, with just over half the egg's total protein.

The average yolk contains 55 calories, all the egg's fat, and just under half of its protein. The yolk also contains a higher amount of vitamins than the white,, including a higher proportion of B_6, B_{12}, folic acid, pantothenic acid, thiamin, calcium, copper, iron, manganese, phosphorus, selenium, and zinc. The yolk also contains all of the vitamins A, D, E, and K.

A large egg is relatively low in fat when you consider the protein and nutrients packed into the shell. With less than 5 grams of fat, one third is saturated fat (1.6 grams) and two thirds is unsaturated (2.8 grams). An egg also contains about 186 milligrams of cholesterol.

Eggs naturally contain small amounts of omega-3 fatty acids. The addition of omega-3 to the hen feed increases the omega-3 fatty acid, which is then passed on to the eggs. Because these amounts are not standardized, there's no way of knowing how much omega-3 the egg you select contains. Eggs advertised as having omega-3 can contain a range between 100 and 600mg. Regular eggs contain only about 30mg per egg.

The Harvard School of Public health states whole egg consumption as part of a healthy diet is acceptable for individuals with low risk of heart disease and normal cholesterol levels. Intake should remain at 1 egg or less per day, including those contained in baked goods. If you have heart disease or high cholesterol levels, it's advisable to limit the amount of dietary cholesterol to less than 200mg per day with a limit of no more than three egg yolks a week. Egg whites may be eaten freely.

 FOODIE FACTOID

Eggs should be stored in the refrigerator at or below 45°F to reduce the risk of food-borne illness. Eggs should never be stored in the door of the refrigerator.

According to the American Egg Board, here are the following are storage times for eggs and egg products:

- Raw eggs in shells: 3-5 weeks
- Raw egg whites: up to 4 days
- Raw egg yolks: up to 4 days
- Hard-boiled eggs: 1 week
- Opened egg substitute: 3 days
- Egg-containing pies and quiches, and egg-based casseroles: 3-4 days
- Commercial eggnog: 3-5 days

Classification of Eggs

Eggs are graded based on height of the white and quality of the yolk. All grades are nutritionally equivalent. Eggs may be Grade AA, A, or B. All eggs sold in retail establishments must be grade B or higher.

Size is based on the weight per dozen of eggs. They may be jumbo, extra large, large, medium, small, or peewee. Most recipes are based on large-sized eggs. The older the hen, the larger the egg will be. The layer's breed also affects the size, as does the weight.

Even though eggs have a fairly long shelf life (in the refrigerator), knowing how fresh your eggs are is important. Eggs may contain three different dates on the carton. The only one required on USDA-graded eggs is called the Julian date—when the eggs are packed. An optional date is the "best by," which must be 45 days or less from the pack date. If "expiration date" is used, the date must be less than 30 days from pack date.

The American Egg Board states the color of the eggshell is not a determinant of how the eggs are raised, its quality, or its nutritional components. The breed of the chicken determines the shell color.

The yolk's color is impacted by the feed. Natural feeds and pigments may change the color of the yolk from bright yellow-orange to pale yellow. Some farmers add natural coloring from flower petals to influence the yolk's color.

Meats

Producers of meat, including beef and pork, are committed to treating all animals humanely, as industries know consumers are concerned about animal rights and care. The farmers and ranchers have a vested interest in keeping animals healthy. To treat animals in any other manner would be self-defeating for farmers and ranchers, as animals fed and cared for properly will be healthier and grow faster.

In addition to the care of animals, global climate change is a concern with all agriculture practices. According to the Environmental Protection Agency (EPA), only 3.4 percent of greenhouse gas emissions are from livestock, and methane from livestock accounts for only 2.8 percent of all world's greenhouse gas emissions. According to the Pork Checkoff Environmental Sustainability Effort, the nation's farmers and ranchers have held their greenhouse gas emissions fairly stable since 1990. This is despite a steady increase in production of almost all animal agricultural products, including an increase of meat by 50 percent, milk by 16 percent, and eggs by 33 percent.

NOTABLE INSIGHT

Commodity checkoff programs collect funds from farmers and producers to provide research and market commodity products. These checkoff programs also provide consumers with information about the specific commodity, including recipes, new uses, nutrition, and safety. Examples of commodity checkoff programs include the American Egg Board, National Pork Board (Pork Checkoff), Cattlemen's Beef Board and National Cattlemen's Beef Association (Beef Checkoff), and the National Dairy Council.

Beef

According to Beef Checkoff, all beef is grass-fed, natural, nutritious, and safe. Variations in raising practices may result in slightly different product labeling, such as grain-finished, grass-finished, naturally raised, and certified organic.

Grain-finished beef cattle spend the majority of their lives grazing on open pastures. The last 4 to 6 months is spent in a feedlot consuming a diet of grains. Grass-finished cattle never spend time in a feedlot but continue grazing pastures. Both grain-finished and grass-finished cattle may be given vitamins and minerals. Antibiotics are administered under careful consideration and only approved growth-promoting hormones are routinely used.

Both naturally raised and certified organic beef may either be grass-finished or grain-finished. Reading the food label can help determine the source of feed the cattle were given the last several months. Certified organic cattle must have 100 percent organic feed if they're grain-finished. Both classifications of beef may be given vitamins and minerals. However, neither may receive antibiotics or growth-promoting hormones, and the USDA must certify both products.

Lean beef is rich in nutrients and can be part of a healthy diet. With high biologically available protein, a 3-ounce portion of lean beef provides 25 grams of protein and 184 calories. Containing about 10 grams of total fat, lean beef is less than half saturated fat. Lean beef is also an excellent source of niacin, B_6, B_{12}, zinc, iron, and selenium.

 NOTABLE INSIGHT

Choosing lean cuts of beef is key in maintaining a heart-healthy diet. The Beef Checkoff offers the following popular lean cuts of beef:

Cut (3-oz. portion)	Calories	Total fat	Sat fat
Top round roast	138	3.2g	1.2g
Sirloin tip steak	148	5.3g	1.9g
Flank steak	158	6.3g	2.6g
Tenderloin steak	168	7.1g	2.8g
Ribeye filet	169	7.8g	2.7g
Ground beef 93% lean	162	7.5g	3.1g
Tri-tip roast	164	8.3g	3.0g

Beef contains primarily monounsaturated and saturated fat. Cattle feed can impact the beef's fatty acid profile. According to the Beef Checkoff, feeding grain for an extended length of time can increase the levels of monounsaturated fat in the end product, which can have a cholesterol-lowering effect. Beef allowed to graze longer on grass will have a higher fatty acid profile. Keeping this in perspective, a 3-ounce portion of grass-finished beef has 0.055g of omega-3 versus 0.02 grams in grain-finished beef. The DRI for omega-3 is 1.1 grams per day for women and 1.6 grams for men.

Pork

Pork farmers have a longstanding relationship with reducing the impact their industry has on the environment. Less than 1 percent of greenhouse gas emissions come from the pork industry, as pigs inherently are not methane producers.

In 2008, pork producers approved a list of ethical principles. U.S. producers accept the responsibility the consumer puts on them to ensure pork products are safe and raised in a humane and ethical manner. These principles include addressing food safety, animal well-being, the animal's environment, public health, employee care, and the communities in which they operate.

Pork products are marketed as "The Other White Meat." According to the Pork Checkoff, lean cuts of pork often have less total fat than skinless chicken breasts and a similar amount of saturated fat. Pork is an excellent source of thiamin, selenium, protein, niacin, vitamin B_6, and phosphorus. Lean cuts of pork, such as loin and chops, are a healthy part of a balanced diet.

NOTABLE INSIGHT

Choosing lean cuts of pork is key in maintaining a heart-healthy diet. The Pork Checkoff recommends the following lean cuts of pork.

Cut (3-oz. portion)	Calories	Total fat	Sat fat
Tenderloin	120	3.0g	1.0g
New York chop	173	5.2g	1.6g
New York roast	147	5.3g	1.6g
Loin center chop	153	6.2g	1.8g
Pork sirloin roast	173	8.0g	2.4g
Ribeye chop	157	7.1g	2.2g

Fish

Industrial-scale fishing has left over 90 percent of the fisheries overexploited and unable to keep up with consumer demand. As a result, new ways of raising seafood have been developed to take the pressure off the wild supply. Not all countries or operations consider the environment and the end product. Concern over pollutants and mercury contamination leaves many consumers unsure how to make safe selections when it comes to fish.

Endangered Species

Overfishing has depleted many species of fish, causing very low levels remaining in the wild and leaving some species no longer commercially viable. The fishing industry has attempted to regulate itself as to what species can be fished; how much of a species can be removed; when certain species can be fished, where, and by whom. Sometimes species are products of bycatch, which means they're unintentionally caught.

SeafoodWatch states some countries have set fishing regulations to prevent overfishing. The programs set forth by countries like the United States, Australia, New Zealand, and the Falkland Islands have allowed for species to regenerate their numbers and prevent drastic reductions.

As a consumer, there are ways you can make a difference, such as purchasing only sustainable seafood. Check out sustainable sources of fish before you make your purchase. Visit BlueOcean.com or SeafoodWatch.org or use their app to find sustainable sources of fish before you make a purchase. Look for sustainable fishery logos, or ask where the seafood at your local market comes from.

Fish Farming

The aquaculture industry accounts for over 50 percent of the world's edible fish, and it may actually save the world's fish supply. Over 100 different species are currently being farmed. Each species, farming method, and farm location has its own impact on the marine ecosystem. According to the Monterey Bay Aquarium (operators of SeafoodWatch.org), sustainable fish farming protects the fish's natural habitat by limiting damage and disease, the escape of nonwild fish, and promotes the feeding practices of using wild fish as feed.

Often these aquaculture practices also improve the environment in which they operate. According to SeaWeb, fish farms take the pressure off wild fish resources, allowing wild species to regenerate. Fish farms may actually also help improve the water quality in some areas. Some species remove excess nitrogen in water, which would be used as food for algae blooms. Farms must also maintain standards to ensure waste and diseases are contained.

 FOODIE FACTOID

An example of U.S. farm-raised sustainable seafood is catfish. Farmed catfish are not given hormones, and as with other agriculture practices, antibiotics are only given judiciously. Farm-raised catfish follow environmentally sustainable practices and are endorsed by the Monterey Bay Aquarium, National Audubon Society, and Environmental Defense. According to the Catfish Institute, over 10,000 people are employed in the catfish farming industry in Alabama, Mississippi, Arkansas, and Louisiana. The industry contributes over $4 billion dollars to each state's economy.

Mercury

Methylmercury (mercury) in seafood has also been an ongoing public health concern. Recommendations for types and amounts of seafood containing mercury have changed over the years. Current mercury levels listed only take into account the mercury in fish and not the selenium amounts.

Selenium is an antioxidant and works with vitamins C and E to protect our body against free radicals. One of the biggest sources of selenium in our diet is seafood. Selenium is also an essential component of an amino acid our body makes called selenocysteine. If mercury is present, it irreversibly binds to the selenium, making it unavailable to synthesize the amino acid in the body. Mercury can also bind to the selenium in the selenocysteine amino acid, making it unusable by the body.

According to the Energy and Environmental Research Center, selenium's ability to counteract mercury toxicity has been known since the 1960s. The key is the selenium-to-mercury ratio. If more selenium is consumed than mercury, the mercury binds to what it requires and leaves the excess selenium available for selenoprotein synthesis. If more mercury is consumed than selenium, there's no selenium left after mercury has bound it. This is when problems occur.

Because ocean fish are an excellent source of selenium, mercury amounts in most fish are inconsequential. When seafood is higher in selenium than mercury, all mercury will be bound and rendered ineffective.

Consuming fish is an important way to get heart-healthy fatty acids in your diet. Each serving of 4 to 6 ounces should be about the size of the palm of your hand. According to the Safina Center, women who are breastfeeding or pregnant should eat only fish low in mercury. Children under the age of 12 should consume only 1 ounce for every 20 pounds of body weight.

Coffee

Coffee is a major source of caffeine, which is a stimulant to the central nervous system. Caffeine doesn't stay in the blood, but rather immediately passes into our brain. Caffeine found in coffee is known to raise blood pressure and increase the fight-or-flight stress response. Is coffee healthy for us? Should we be drinking it?

According to AARP, 83 percent of Americans drink coffee on a regular basis. Coffee has been shown to increase mental alertness and help prevent some forms of cancer and stroke. Coffee consumption may also help reduce your chances of developing dementia or Parkinson's disease as well as reduce your risk of cardiovascular disease and type 2 diabetes, according to the U.S. 2015 Dietary Guidelines Advisory Committee.

This committee considers three to five cups per day as moderate coffee consumption. Their research review stated that up to five cups of coffee (400mg of caffeine) per day can provide many health benefits. The key is moderate consumption. The committee also advises that about one cup of coffee (100mg of caffeine) can negatively affect your sleep when consumed around bedtime.

FOODIE FACTOID

Coffee comes from the Arabic word meaning "wine of the bean." Though its roots are in Ethiopia, coffee is enjoyed throughout the world.

The Good News About Your Cup of Joe

The coffee bean is a type of seed. Seeds in general are packed with a variety of nutrients and phytochemicals. According to the Mayo Clinic, no studies as of this date have looked at the antioxidant properties of coffee after it has been brewed and entered our bodies.

In a Japanese study, researchers found that women drinking two to three cups of coffee daily had reduced systemic oxidative DNA damage, which is linked to the formation of cancer cells. Researchers also surmised that habitual coffee consumption reduced the study participants' iron stores and thus decreased the systemic oxidative DNA damage.

The National Cancer Institute (NCI) reports that individuals who consume coffee on a regular basis may have a reduced risk of death. A study conducted by the NCI and AARP showed habitual coffee drinkers were not as likely to die from respiratory disease, heart disease, stroke, injuries, accidents, and infections as their noncoffee-drinking counterparts. This study found equal results for regular coffee and decaffeinated, supporting the hypothesis that phytochemicals in the coffee are likely the beneficial components.

The Alzheimer's Drug Discovery Foundation reports coffee consumption of three to five cups a day, from midlife on, has been linked to a reduced and/or delayed onset of Alzheimer's disease and dementia. When the caffeine in coffee goes straight to the brain, it blocks a type of receptor important in the inflammation response. By blocking the receptor, the chain of events causing the cognitive decline is stopped. The foundation does caution, if the excessive caffeine intake affects sleep causing insomnia, a reduction in cognitive decline may not be experienced.

Harvard Health reports high intake of coffee may slow the onset of type 2 diabetes. However, in type 2 diabetics, consumption of three to six cups of coffee a day may adversely affect blood sugar levels.

Caffeine and Coffee—the Dark Side

Caffeine is addictive. High consumption of caffeine is associated with an increase in anxiety, insomnia. Caffeine may interact with some medications, so please check with your doctor or pharmacist before consuming.

Caffeine has also been shown to have a detrimental effect on your bones. A study published in the *Journal of Nutrition* reports that consuming more than 300mg per day or drinking three or more cups of coffee a day is linked to the inability to absorb sufficient calcium, which has been attributed to bone loss. Younger women who consume adequate calcium may not experience negative results from caffeine. However, it's recommended that older women increase calcium intake when consuming caffeine.

NOTABLE INSIGHT

Be aware of how much caffeine you're consuming from your daily coffee. The USDA National Nutrient Database lists the following amounts of caffeine in various coffee drinks:

- Espresso (1 oz.): 40-75mg
- Instant coffee (8 oz.): 27-173mg
- Brewed coffee (8 oz.): 95-200mg
- Brewed decaf coffee (8 oz.): 2-13mg
- McDonald's brewed coffee (16 oz.): 100mg
- Starbuck's brewed coffee (16 oz.): 330mg
- Specialty espresso beverage such as latte (8 oz.): 63-175mg

A Swiss study shows the consumption of decaffeinated coffee in individuals who do not regularly drink it increased blood pressure and muscle sympathetic nerve activity. The researchers believe there are components in the coffee other than just the caffeine that may attribute to cardiovascular changes. In fact, sympathetic nerve activity (the fight-or-flight response) reaches its peak about 60 minutes after consumption. In nonhabitual coffee drinkers, blood pressure significantly increased. There wasn't a significant effect on the blood pressure of those individuals who regularly drink coffee.

Coffee is one of the most common stomach irritants, as it's very acidic and irritates the GI tract easily. Individuals with heartburn and gastroesophageal reflux disease (GERD) should avoid all coffee, even decaffeinated, which has been shown to be even more irritating to the stomach for some than regular coffee. Caffeine, in addition to coffee itself, can induce acid reflux by relaxing the muscles in your GI tract, allowing the contents to back up into your esophagus.

According to Harvard Health, there are substances in coffee, cafestol and kahweol, that can raise your LDL cholesterol. These two substances are oily and can be easily filtered out with paper filters. They are found in Turkish coffee, coffee made with a French press, boiled coffee, and espresso. However, cafestol and kahweol are not filtered out of espresso.

Wine

There are many negative health consequences associated with alcohol and its addictive properties. However, people have been making wine for eons, and many of those large populations that consume it on a regular basis tend to be healthier and live longer.

Polyphenols (antioxidant components) found in wine along with flavonoids have been shown to reduce the risk of heart disease by lowering LDL cholesterol and raising HDL. The key, however, is drinking it only in moderation.

Moderate consumption of alcohol means no than one (5-ounce) glass a day for all women and men over 65 years of age and no more than two glasses a day for men under the age of 65. Excessive alcohol has many negative health consequences. The American Heart Association (AHA) doesn't recommend starting to drink alcohol, however, simply to prevent disease.

Researchers aren't sure if all alcoholic beverages, including beer and liquor, are as beneficial to the heart as wine is. The Mayo Clinic reports that researchers have discovered drinking any alcohol, not just red wine, can have health benefits, too. Alcohol may increase HDL cholesterol, reduce the chance of blood clots, and reduce damage done by LDL cholesterol.

Health Benefits

Resveratrol, an antioxidant found in the skins of grapes, is the reason red wine became known for its health benefits. Red wine grapes spend more time with the skins attached than white wine grapes due to longer fermenting time, and this appears to have a beneficial affect. However, it's now thought that white wine may have similar benefits to red wine as well.

The Mayo Clinic reports much of the research done on the health benefits of red wine and resveratrol has been done on animals. The results have been promising, showing benefits relating to reducing obesity, heart disease, and diabetes. However, these results have not been duplicated in humans and amounts for human intake to reach the same levels as animals would be equivalent to drinking 1,000 liters of wine each day!

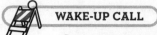

WAKE-UP CALL

Some consumers wanting the health benefits of resveratrol are turning to supplements to get the recommended does of 1,000-1,500mg per day from a pill. Remember, supplements are not regulated, so choose brands that have been voluntarily audited. Always discuss your supplement usage with your medical providers. Note that resveratrol has anticoagulant properties, and it may interfere with blood thinners such as Coumadin or Warfarin.

Supplements, grape juice, and other foods containing resveratrol like blueberries, cranberries, and peanuts may be options for obtaining its health benefits without consuming alcohol.

The AHA states that middle-aged men and women are at a greater risk of heart disease and also would benefit the most from light to moderate wine consumption. Moderate wine intake of one or two glasses a day or three to four a week is associated with a 30 percent reduced likelihood of developing plaque deposits on artery walls.

Breast Cancer Risk

Alcohol intake has also been shown to increase the risk of certain types of breast cancer. Hormones like estrogen are increased by the ingestion of alcohol. When alcohol is broken down in the body, it forms acetaldehyde. This component has the ability to damage cellular DNA and proteins in the body.

The American Cancer Society reports an increase of 10 to 12 percent risk for every drink a woman consumes. The National Cancer Institute reports that women who drink the equivalent of three drinks per day have a 1.5 greater risk to develop breast cancer. Increased alcohol intake also increases risk of developing other forms of cancer.

Beer

Beer contains as many antioxidants as wine, but they're different due to the ingredients that go into the making of beer, specifically barley and hops. Beer has more protein and B vitamins than wine. Research has shown all alcoholic beverages are likely as good as the next in preventing heart disease. Beer, in moderation, has many health benefits. Remember, though, it is still alcohol.

A report published in *Nature* states the yeast found in beer acts as a prebiotic in your gut. Common gut microbes break down yeast to use as energy. Healthy bacteria in your gut translates it to a healthy gut overall.

According to the *Beer and Wine Journal*, ferulic acid is found in beer and is bound to the malt. If the mashed grains are allowed to rest during beer making, the ferulic acid is released from the malt. An increase in ferulic acid in turn increases the amount of 4VG molecules, and these molecules give beer made from wheat or wheat malt its distinct aroma.

 WAKE-UP CALL

For over 100 years, doctors prescribed Guinness to pregnant women for the added B vitamins. We now know drinking alcohol during pregnancy can cause harm to the fetus. According to the USDA National Nutrient Database, beer does contain some B vitamins, but the quantities are less than 1 percent of the DRI.

The National Institutes of Health (NIH) states ferulic acid has many possible health benefits. With regular consumption, this powerful antioxidant may help protect against oxidative stress. Ferulic acid has the highest bioavailability of the flavonoid class of polyphenols. Multiple derivatives of the acid have been linked to cancer prevention, diabetes prevention, and antiaging treatment, as well as possible protective qualities for liver and neurodegenerative disease. This ferulic acid is a powerful antioxidant and may help prevent inflammation.

The Least You Need to Know

- Eggs are an excellent source of protein and contain many vitamins and minerals that are part of a healthy diet.
- Selecting the right cuts of meat and eating the proper serving size can help you achieve healthy results.
- You can support sustainable seafood practices by choosing the safe species of fish.
- Research shows that coffee can offer some health benefits, but it should be consumed in moderation.
- Drinking alcohol is a personal decision, and you should consider your individual health risks before consumption.

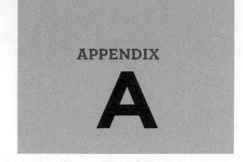

APPENDIX

A

Glossary

% Daily Value (%DV)   A recommendation for key nutrients that is based on a 2,000-calorie diet.

acceptable macronutrient distribution range (AMDR)   A recommended range of percentage of intakes for carbohydrates, protein, and fats to help ensure people get enough healthy nutrients in their diets while limiting others to help ward off disease.

acid reflux   When stomach contents move backwards up into the esophagus.

amino acids   The building blocks of proteins.

amylase   The enzyme contained in your saliva that acts on the food in its moistened state, which begins breaking down starches.

anaphylaxis   A severe and life-threatening reaction that affects the whole body, usually occurring within seconds or minutes after exposure to an allergen.

angina   A reduction in adequate blood flow that can result pain in the chest, shoulders, neck, arms, jaw, or back, and is caused by plaque buildup in arteries.

anorexia   An eating disorder in which a person eats too little food to maintain a healthy weight.

anthocyanidins   Includes the dietary flavonoids cyanidin, delphinidin, malvidin, pelargonidin, peonidin, and petunidin, which are responsible for the red, blue, and purple pigments found in plants.

antioxidants   Plant chemicals that protect your cells from damage from free radicals, which are produced during normal cell metabolism.

asymptomatic allergy   A food allergy that involves antibodies but doesn't always produce symptoms.

atherosclerosis   The buildup of fats, cholesterol, and other substances causing plaque to form in the artery, which results in restricted blood flow.

basal metabolic rate (BMR)   The total number of calories your body needs at rest.

beta-carotene   A phytonutrient that is also the precursor to vitamin A.

binge-eating disorder (BED)   A disorder characterized by consuming large amounts of food in a very short period of time.

bioavailability   Refers to an active chemical compound being physiologically available for use in the body.

body dysmorphic disorder (BDD)   A severe form of negative body image in which individuals become obsessed with their perceived flaws.

body mass index (BMI)   A calculation used by many health practitioners to determine if a person is at a healthy weight based on his or her weight-to-height ratio.

bolus   Swallowed food.

bulimia   An eating disorder characterized by repeatedly eating large amounts of foods and then purging those foods with self-induced vomiting or the use of laxatives along with excessive exercise to prevent weight gain.

calorie   A unit of measure to determine the total amount of energy that's provided from proteins, carbohydrates, and fats.

carbohydrate   A macronutrient that provides 4 calories per gram and is classified as either simple or complex.

carbon footprint   Refers to the amount of pressure on the environment related to a particular product or system that's measured by the amount of greenhouse gas emitted.

carotenoids   Phytochemicals, such as lycopene, lutein, and zeaxanthin, that include more than 600 plant pigments and are the primary sources for orange, red, and yellow colors.

catechin   The primary phytonutrient found in tea leaves from the *Camellia sinensis* plant.

celiac disease   An autoimmune disorder of the intestines that results in a person not being able to ingest gluten, a protein found in wheat, rye, and barley.

chlorophyll   A green plant pigment that allows a plant to capture light energy and convert it into plant energy through photosynthesis.

cholecystokinin (CCK)   A hormone released to digest fat and protein, which also informs the brain that it's no longer hungry.

cholesterol   A waxy substance that's present in all the cells in your body.

Clean Fifteen   A list of the 15 produce items that have been tested for the least amount of pesticide residue.

conventional farming   Crops grown with the use of pesticides, synthetic chemical fertilizers, herbicides, and GMOs.

cooperatives (co-ops)   Farms owned and operated by a group of members with a common interest and for the benefit of all members.

coronary artery disease (CAD)   Occurs when the arteries that supply your heart with oxygen, blood, and nutrients become diseased or damaged.

Crohn's disease   An inflammatory bowel disease that causes inflammation in any location throughout the digestive tract.

Dietary Approaches to Stop Hypertension (DASH) diet   A diet designed to lower blood pressure that reduces saturated and trans fats, cholesterol, sodium, and refined sugar.

Dietary Guidelines for Americans   Governmental guidelines published every five years that provide valuable information on what we should be eating and drinking to promote health, maintain our weight, and ward off diseases.

Dirty Dozen   Refers to the top 12 fruits and vegetables that contain the highest amounts of pesticide residue, and that you may want to consider purchasing as organic.

electrolytes   Minerals that aid in the maintenance of your body's fluid balance inside and outside of the cells.

empty calorie food   A food in which the majority of calories are from sugars or fats and that doesn't provide any additional vitamins or minerals.

environmental working group (EWG)   A nonprofit, independent group that conducts random pesticide residue testing on fruits and vegetables.

epiglottis   The flap of cartilage that covers the trachea and prevents food from going down into your windpipe.

fad diets   Diets that are a temporary fix to a lifelong problem, which can lead to nutritional deficiencies, metabolic issues, and muscle loss.

fat-soluble vitamins   Includes vitamins A, D, E, and K, which are stored in the liver or fatty tissues.

flavonoids   A large group of phytonutrients that are categorized as polyphenolic compounds, which aid in cell-signaling pathways dealing with cell growth and death.

fluid balance   Balance is achieved when the amount of fluid taken in equals the amount of fluid lost from the body.

food additive   A manmade or natural product added to a food that doesn't contain it in its original state.

food allergy   Occurs when the body mistakes certain food proteins as harmful and mounts an immunologic attack by producing antibodies, histamines, and other defensive mechanisms as protection.

food intolerance   Occurs when there's a reaction to a food that doesn't involve an immune system response.

food sensitivity   A non-IgE allergy response that involves an immune response.

functional fiber   Refers to isolated, purified forms of nondigestible carbohydrates that have beneficial effects in humans and are made from fiber extracted from plants or animals.

genetically modified organisms (GMOs)   Organisms created when selected genes from one organism are inserted into the DNA of another, thus altering the organism's DNA.

glycemic index (GI)   A measurement of how much each gram of available carbohydrate (total carbohydrate minus fiber) in a single serving of a food affects your blood glucose level.

high-density lipoprotein (HDL)   Considered the "good" cholesterol, HDL is made up of high-density lipoproteins and is a combination of 50 percent protein, 20 percent cholesterol, phospholipid, and triglyceride molecules.

hydrogenation   The process of heating liquid oil under pressure while exposing it to hydrogen gas and a catalyst to create a lab-made trans fat.

hypertension   High blood pressure.

hyponatremia   A condition in which the sodium in the blood is lower than normal.

immune response   How the body recognizes and defends itself against bacteria, viruses, and substances that appear foreign and harmful.

immunoglobulin E (IgE)   Antibodies that are directed to initiate a chemical release within certain cells, which then produce an allergic reaction in the body.

inflammatory bowel disease (IBD)   A general term for illnesses that result from a frequent immune response and chronic inflammation of the gastrointestinal tract.

insoluble fiber   Fiber that doesn't dissolve in water and adds bulk to the foodstuff in your GI tract. This fiber keeps nutrients moving through your system by adding roughage, decreasing transit time, and making it easier for you to go to the bathroom.

insulin resistance   Occurs when the body can produce insulin without a problem but cannot utilize it effectively.

intrinsic factor   An essential glycoprotein that's produced by the parietal cells within the stomach in order for the body to efficiently absorb vitamin B12.

irritable bowel syndrome (IBS)   A functional GI disorder that causes the digestive tract to perform in an irregular way without evidence of damage to the digestive tract.

isoflavones   Phytonutrients that are water-soluble and heat-stable and include the flavonoids daidzein, genistein, and glycitein.

ketogenesis   The breakdown of fat due to an inadequate supply of carbohydrates.

large intestine   Also referred to as the colon.

leaky gut syndrome   Occurs when there's increased permeability within the intestines due to a microflora imbalance.

leptin   A hormone produced from adipocytes or fat cells in your body that signals the brain when your fat stores are low.

Lifestyle Eating and Performance (LEAP)   An effective protocol that combines the Mediator Release Test (MRT) with the skills of a Certified LEAP Therapist to produce a patient-specific diet.

locavore   A person who consumes foods grown locally, generally within a 100-mile radius.

low-density lipoprotein (LDL)   Considered "bad" cholesterol, LDL is made up of 50 percent cholesterol, phospholipid, triglycerides, and 25 percent protein molecules.

lower digestive tract   Refers to the small and large intestines.

lycopene   A plant pigment that makes vegetables and fruits red and belongs to the group of carotenoids.

major minerals   The set of minerals required by the body in amounts of more than 100mg per day. These include calcium, magnesium, sodium, phosphorus, sulfate, potassium, and chloride.

malabsorption syndrome   The direct result of another disease or disorder that causes the intestines to not properly absorb certain nutrients.

Mediator Release Test (MRT)   A simple blood test that measures your immune reaction or sensitivity to a whole host of foods and also food additives and chemicals.

meditation   A practice that has been used for centuries to help find inner peace and deal with life stresses.

microvilli   Hairlike projections found in the intestines that contain digestive enzymes from the mucosa cells in the lining.

minerals   Inorganic elements that don't contain carbon and occur naturally in soil and water.

monounsatured fat   Fat molecules with one unsaturated carbon bond. Oils that contain these types of fats are liquid at room temperature, solidify when chilled, and are considered to be heart healthy.

neurotransmitters   Chemicals responsible for sending communication signals throughout your body. They can either stimulate the brain or calm the brain. Stress, poor diet, genetics, drugs, alcohol, and caffeine adversely affect these levels.

omega-3 fatty acids   Polyunsaturated fatty acids that are essential. Commonly found in fatty fishes such as salmon, mackerel, tuna, herring, sardines, anchovies, and trout.

omega-6 fatty acids   Polyunsaturated fatty acids that are essential. They're commonly found in safflower oil, walnut oil, sunflower oil, corn oil, and soybean oil.

oral allergy syndrome   Occurs due to cross-reacting allergens in pollen, raw fruits and vegetables, and some tree nuts. Symptoms include a tingling, itching, or swelling of the lips, tongue, and throat.

organic   Products that are created with concern for the environment and without use of antibiotics, growth hormones, GMOs, pesticides, and synthetic fertilizers.

Organic System Plan   Also known as the Farm Plan, this system helps farms improve management and conserve and optimize resources, and is a legal contract between the producer and certifying agency.

orthorexia   When a person has an obsession with eating "healthy" foods.

oxidative damage   An imbalance between the body's ability to detoxify the harmful effects of free radicals and their rate of production.

Oxygen Radical Absorbance Capacity (ORAC)   A scale for foods that measures the total antioxidant capacity of a particular food in a test tube and its ability to prevent oxidation by free radicals.

peer review process   A collaborative process in which an author's work or research is evaluated and commented on by peers in their field.

peptic ulcer   Occurs when stomach acids that digest food cause erosion in the stomach wall or duodenum.

peripheral artery disease (PAD)   A condition when arteries become narrow and restrict blood flow to the limbs.

phytonutrient   Plant nutrients that offer the body a protective health benefit and help ward off disease.

polyphenols Phytonutrients that act as powerful antioxidants and are found in many foods in our diet.

polyunsaturated fat Fat molecules that have more than one double bond. Oils that contain these fats are liquid at room temperature and don't typically solidify when chilled.

prebiotics Nondigestible carbohydrates, such as plant fiber, that assist in the growth of existing bacteria in the colon.

probiotics Healthy bacteria and yeast found in yogurt or kefer and that also can be taken as a supplement.

protein A macronutrient that provides 4 calories per gram and plays a very important role in the development, maintenance, and repair of the human body.

registered dietitian nutritionist (RDN) A professional who has studied the science of nutrition and practical solutions for health.

satiety The feeling of fullness after eating.

saturated fat A type of fat that's solid at room temperature and primarily comes from animal products such as dairy, red meat, and poultry that should only be consumed in limited amounts.

sickle cell anemia A genetic blood disorder that affects red blood cells and causes them to form in a crescent shape instead of being round.

simple carbohydrates Monosaccharaides that include glucose, fructose, and galactose.

small intestine The primary site of nutrient digestion and absorption. It's composed of three sections—the duodenum, jejunum, and ileum.

soluble fiber Fiber that dissolves in water and forms a gel, and also slows down digestion and makes you feel full.

sphincter A circular muscle portal between key passages in the GI tract that controls the release of food.

trace minerals Minerals required by the body in amounts less than 20mg per day, including iron, iodine, chromium, molybdenum, copper, zinc, fluoride, selenium, and manganese.

trans fat A fat that occurs naturally in small amounts in beef, lamb, and butterfat, or is made artificially in a lab and found in processed foods and is no longer recognized as safe by the Food and Drug Administration (FDA).

triglyceride The primary storage form for fats in your body. A high level of triglycerides can harden your arteries and increase the risk of heart disease and stroke, along with contributing to obesity and metabolic syndrome.

type 2 diabetes   A metabolic disorder in which the body is unable to produce enough insulin and/or use it effectively.

ulcerative colitis   An inflammatory bowel disease that causes sores and inflammation within the lining of the colon and rectum.

upper digestive tract   Refers to the oral cavity, esophagus, and stomach.

vitamins   Naturally occurring organic compounds that are required by the body for nutrition and growth.

water-soluble vitamins   These vitamins include all of the B vitamins and vitamin C, can be dissolved in water, and are not stored in the body.

xanthoma   A skin condition where cholesterol-rich material is deposited under the surface of the skin. It's most commonly associated with medical conditions that increase blood lipids, such as hyperlipidemia, diabetes, and pancreatitis.

Online Resources

The following online resources will help further your knowledge and keep you up to date. This information was reliable and correct at the time of this writing; we assume no responsibility for any recent changes in the contact information that may have occurred since the initial printing of this book.

Websites for Further Reading

Health Organizations

Academy of Nutrition and Dietetics
eatright.org

American Cancer Society
cancer.org

American Heart Association
heart.org

Centers for Disease Control and Prevention
cdc.gov

Consumerlab
consumerlab.com

Cleveland Clinic
my.clevelandclinic.org

Environmental Protection Agency
epa.gov

Food Allergy Research & Education
foodallergy.org

Harvard School of Public Health
hsph.harvard.edu

Institute of Medicine
iom.nationalacademies.org

Mayo Clinic
mayoclinic.org

National Cancer Institute
cancer.gov

National Institutes of Health
nih.gov

National Institute of Neurological Disorders and Stroke
ninds.nih.gov

National Sleep Foundation
sleepfoundation.org

Office of Disease Prevention and Health Promotion
health.gov

U.S. Department of Health & Human Services
hhs.gov

U.S. Department of Agriculture
usda.gov

USDA ChooseMyPlate.gov
choosemyplate.gov

U.S. Food and Drug Administration
fda.gov

Food

American Egg Board
aeb.org

Beef Checkoff
beefitswhatsfordinner.com

Food and Agriculture Organization of the United Nations
fao.org

Mediterranean Foods Alliance's Oldways Program
mediterraneanmark.org

National Dairy Council
nationaldairycouncil.org

The Nature Conservancy
nature.org

The Olive Oil Source
oliveoilsource.com

Pork Checkoff
porkandhealth.org

Produce for Better Health Foundation
pbhfoundation.org

Safina Center
safinacenter.org

Seafood Watch by Monterey Bay Aquarium
seafoodwatch.org

USDA Farmers Markets
search.ams.usda.gov/farmersmarkets

Whole Grains Council
wholegrainscouncil.org

Support

Am I Hungry?
amihungry.com

National Eating Disorders Association
nationaleatingdisorders.org

Overeaters Anonymous
Overeatersanonymous.org

Index

molybdenum, 132
monoglycerides, 96
monosaccharides, 73
monosodium glutamate (MSG), 161, 174
monounsaturated fats, 20, 98, 276
  chemical structure, 98
  consumption, 181
  health benefits of, 98, 180
  percentage of in cooking oils, 181
mood, food and, 34-35
mood disorders, 37
  cognitive decline, 39
  depression, 38
  seasonal affective disorder, 38
  serotonin sensitive disorders, 40
  zinc levels, 38
mRNA. *See* messenger RNA
MRT. *See* Mediator Release Test
MSG. *See* monosodium glutamate
multiple sclerosis, 50

N

National Association of Anorexia Nervosa and Associated Disorders, 207, 209
National Cancer Institute (NCI), 289
National Eating Disorder Association, 208
National Health and Nutrition Examination Survey (NHANES), 66
National Institute of Medicine (NIM), 174
National Sleep Foundation, 35
natural ingredients, 173
NCGS. *See* non-celiac gluten sensitivity

NCI. *See* National Cancer Institute
neural tube defects, 116
neuropeptide Y, 205
neurotransmitters, 40, 84, 199
NHANES. *See* National Health and Nutrition Examination Survey
niacin (B3), 114
NIM. *See* National Institute of Medicine
NLEA. *See* Nutrition Labeling and Education Act
non-celiac gluten sensitivity (NCGS), 220
nonheme iron, 130, 256
nonhydrogenated shortening, 189
non-IgE allergy, 219
nonnutritive sweeteners, 76
nonsteroidal anti-inflammatory drugs, 24
nutrition facts label, 160
nutritionists, 11
Nutrition Labeling and Education Act (NLEA), 160

O

oatmeal, 133, 153
obesity, 15
  choices leading to, 15
  epidemic, 9
  fad diets, 17
  hazard foods, 16
  risk of, 16
  sleep and, 36
  solution foods, 17
  triglycerides and, 100
obsessive-compulsive disorder (OCD), 40
OCD. *See* obsessive-compulsive disorder

oleoresins, 173
oligosaccharides, 77
olive oil, 180, 182-183
omega-3 fatty acids, 18, 99, 105
  benefits of, 275
  blood pressure and, 22
  fish as source of, 158
  salmon as source of, 274
  vegetarian diets, 256
  walnuts as source of, 276
omega-6s, 100
oral allergy syndrome, 220
organic products, 169
  beef, 285
  eggs, 282
  labeling, 170
Organic System Plan, 172
orthorexia, 69
osmosis, 126
osteoarthritis, 139
osteomalacia, 120, 126
osteoporosis, 92, 126, 143, 257
ovarian cancer, 139
overeating, protein deficiency and, 91
ovo-vegetarians, 256
oxalates, 124
oxidative damage, 132

P

packaging claims, 162
  health claims, 164-165
  nutrient claims, 162
  regulation, 163
  relative nutrient claims, 163
  structure and function claims, 165
PAD. *See* peripheral artery disease
Paleolithic diet, 262-263
palm oil, 188

Q-R